Pet Owner Educational Atlas

DENTISTRY AND ORAL SURGERY

Texts and review: Aurora Mateo Román

edra
PUBLISHING

This book was originally published in Spanish under the title:
Atlas de información al propietario. Odontología y cirugía oral

ISBN Spanish edition: 978-84-18020-44-5

Pet Owner Educational Atlas. Dentistry and Oral Surgery
Aurora Mateo Román

ISBN: 978-1-962679-30-5

Publishing Manager: Costanza Smeraldi, Edra S.p.A.
Paper, Printing and Binding Manager: Paolo Ficicchia, Edra S.p.A.
Cover, Layout, Translation and Copyediting: Grupo Asís Biomedia S.L.

Edra Publishing US LLC
3309 Northlake Boulevard, Suite 203
Palm Beach Gardens, FL, 33403
EIN: 844113980
info@edrapublishing.com
www.edrapublishing.com

edra
PUBLISHING

Printed in Italy by GALLI & C. – Gavirate (VA)
January 2025

PREFACE

Firstly, I would like to thank the publisher for its initiative in dedicating a volume of the Pet Owner Educational Atlas series to the specialty of dentistry and oral surgery in cats and dogs. I would also like to thank Lisa Milella, my mentor, for her invaluable support during my residency and in the preparation of this work.

Pet owners are increasingly demanding more effective and painless treatments, and veterinary dentistry is gradually ceasing to be a difficult and little-known specialty. This book provides the tools required to educate owners on the importance of an early diagnosis, given that pets do not "talk" and it is our responsibility to learn to detect their discomfort as soon as possible. Of course, to achieve this, the collaboration and participation of owners is of vital importance. Pets with dental pathologies usually do not lose their appetites, and owners do not typically detect if their pet is suffering from oral discomfort or pain. Because of this, pets sometimes have to endure a greater or lesser degree of "pain" and "infection" for months or even years until they are finally treated.

Some of these pathologies can be easily identified in the consultation room, with the animal conscious, but, in most cases, the definitive diagnosis and true extent of the disease can only be detected under general anesthesia.

Here, a complete data collection system (odontogram) is provided to help professionals learn how to write dental reports, file relevant clinical information, and tell owners what specific problem their pet has and what type of treatment should be implemented.

Each pathology is explained in a simple way, with drawings based on real cases and accompanied by the different treatment options available. Veterinarians can draw on the sheets to help them convey their message to pet owners. I am convinced that this new atlas will be as useful for clinicians as it is for me in my daily work.

Aurora Mateo, DVM

FOREWORD

Dental and oral diseases are among the most common disorders in companion animals. They also affect wild animals both in the wild and in captivity and have important consequences on animal health and welfare when undiagnosed and untreated. However, these diseases are still frequently underestimated. The lack of university programs that include training in veterinary dentistry is a global problem that affects even the most developed countries.

Fortunately, awareness of animal welfare in this sense has increased in recent years. Training options in veterinary dentistry are becoming more frequent. Veterinary practitioners are also more aware of the need for training, both in basic dental diagnosis and treatment and in the detection of pathologies that require referral to a specialist. Working together with veterinary dentists, clinicians can provide their patients with a standard of quality in animal welfare in accordance with modern veterinary clinical practice.

I have had the pleasure of learning about Aurora's enormous body of work and of mentoring her during her residency at the European Veterinary Dental College. This book is the product of her experience and I am sure that it will contribute to the development of this specialty, increasing the interest of veterinary clinicians in veterinary dentistry, both in terms of identification and diagnosis and in providing their clients with an adequate explanation of the various treatment options.

The best reward will be the owner's satisfaction at seeing an improvement in their pet's quality of life after receiving adequate and effective dental treatment.

Lisa Milella, DEVDC
Founder of The Lisa Milella Veterinary Dental Fund
https://www.internationalanimalrescue.org/lmvdf

Table of contents

01 ANATOMY APPLIED TO DIAGNOSIS

02 PERIODONTAL DISEASE

03 DENTAL PATHOLOGIES

04 ORAL DISEASES AND NEOPLASMS

05 COMMON ORAL PROCEDURES AND DENTAL EMERGENCIES

1 Location terminology

Knowing location terminology is useful in dentistry because teeth are numerous and it is imperative to accurately define the location of any lesion or process. It is especially useful if the case is to be referred.

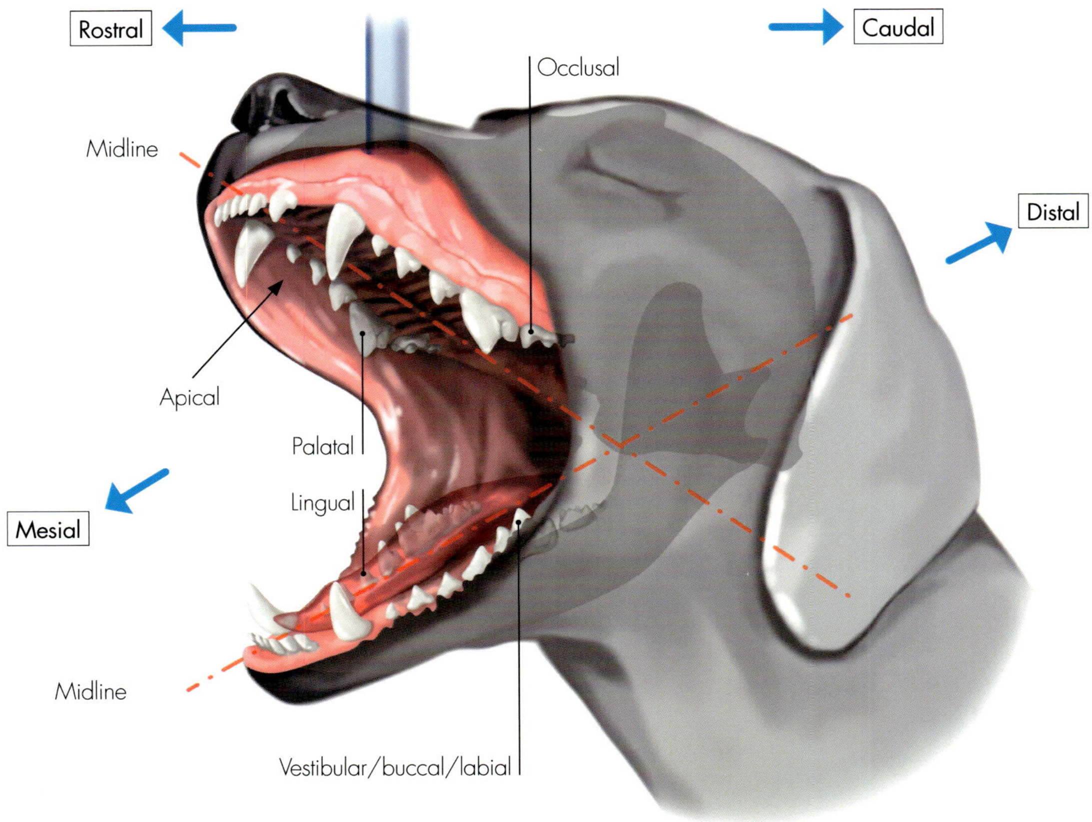

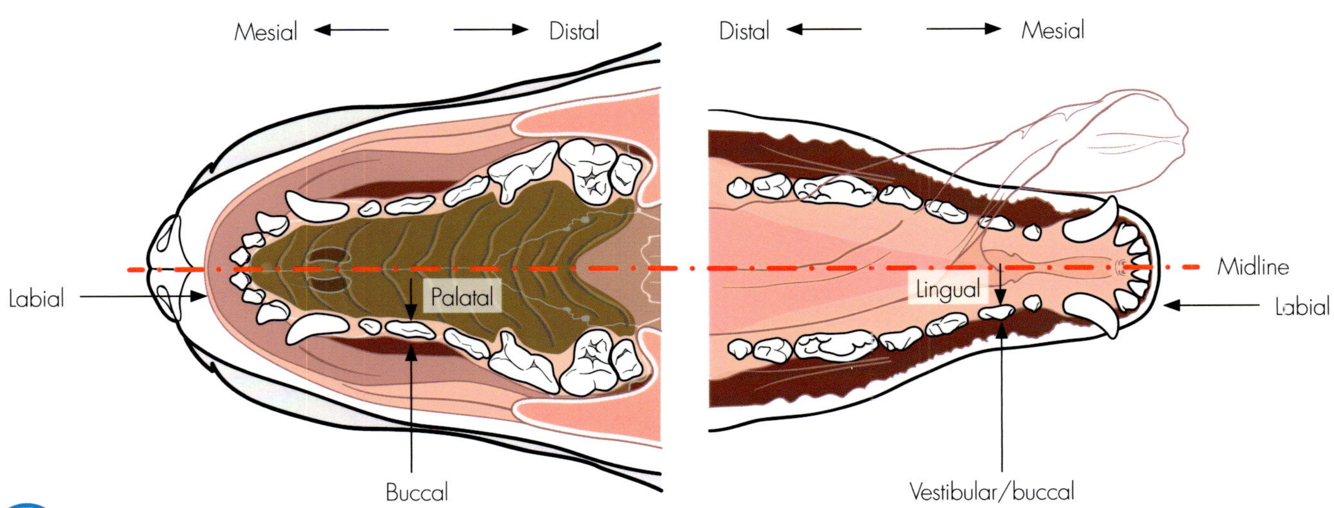

The terms to describe direction are equivalent in cats and dogs.

2 How many teeth do dogs have?

Download a sample odontogram for your use

Teeth are part of the digestive system and perform numerous functions. Cats and dogs are carnivores and their teeth are adapted to killing and cutting prey into pieces that can be swallowed. In addition, the mouth plays an important role to pets as a means of contact and communication with their owners. Dental formulas are used to determine the type and total number of teeth present per quadrant. The upper numbers indicate the maxillary teeth up to the midline, while the lower numbers indicate the same for the mandibular teeth. The set is multiplied by two to obtain the total number of teeth.

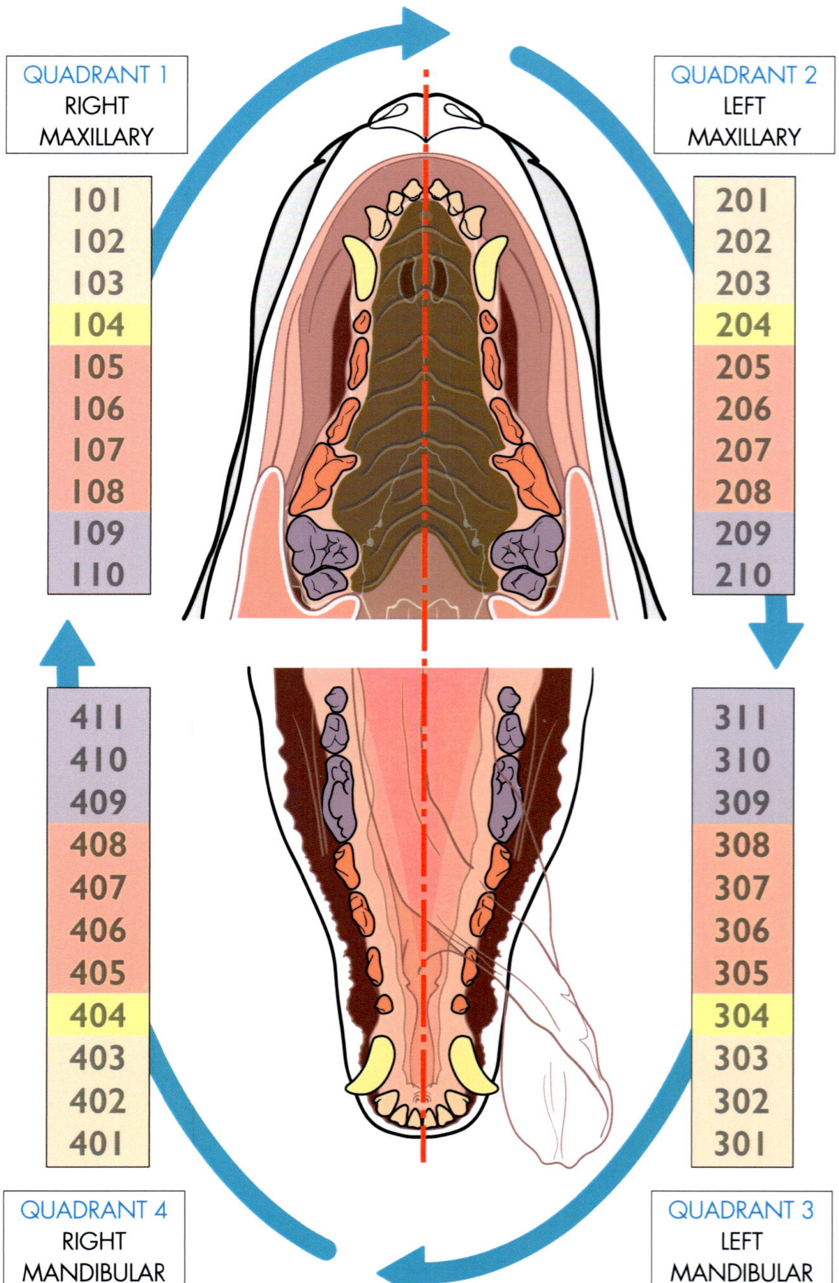

Dental formula

$$2\times(I\,\frac{3}{3}\;C\,\frac{1}{1}\;P\,\frac{4}{4}\;M\,\frac{2}{3}) = 42 \text{ teeth}$$

Number of roots	Maxillary teeth	Mandibular teeth
1	I, C, P1	I, C, P1, M3
2	P2, P3	P2, P3, P4, M1, M2
3	P4, M1, M2	—

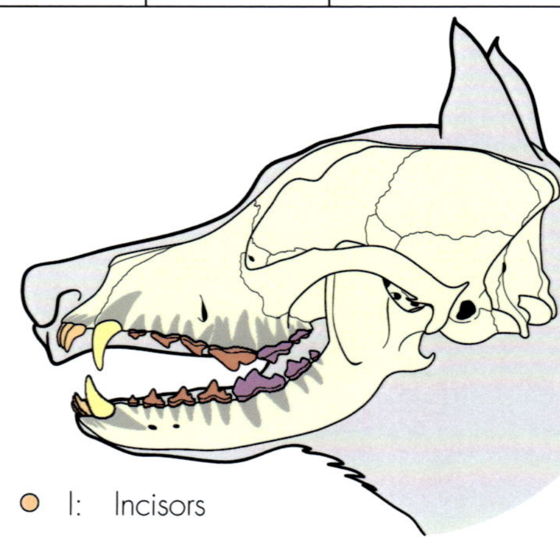

- I: Incisors
- C: Canines
- P: Premolars
- M: Molars

Features

- **Heterodont** teeth: different shape and function.
- **Brachydont** teeth: short crown and relatively longer root.
- **Anelodont** teeth: they reach their developmental potential and do not grow any more.
- **Diphyodont**: animal with two types of dentition, deciduous and permanent.

3 How many teeth do puppies have?

Download a sample odontogram for your use

Cats and dogs have deciduous (milk) teeth that are later replaced with permanent dentition. Milk teeth have their own nomenclature and characteristics, with a different dental formula from that of adults. Nonetheless, it is important to care for the health of the teeth of cats and dogs from the time they are kittens and puppies.

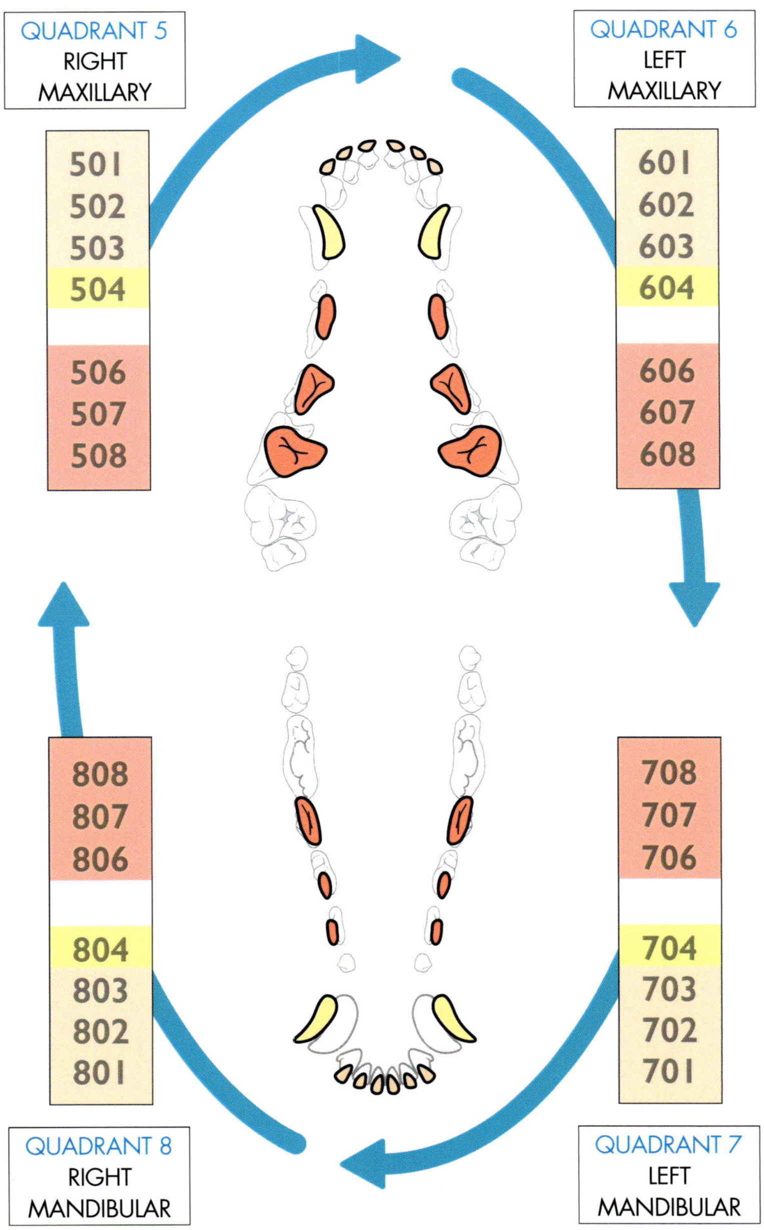

Dental formula

$$2\times\left(i\,\frac{3}{3}\;c\,\frac{1}{1}\;p\,\frac{3}{3}\right) = 28 \text{ teeth}$$

Lowercase letters are used for deciduous dentition

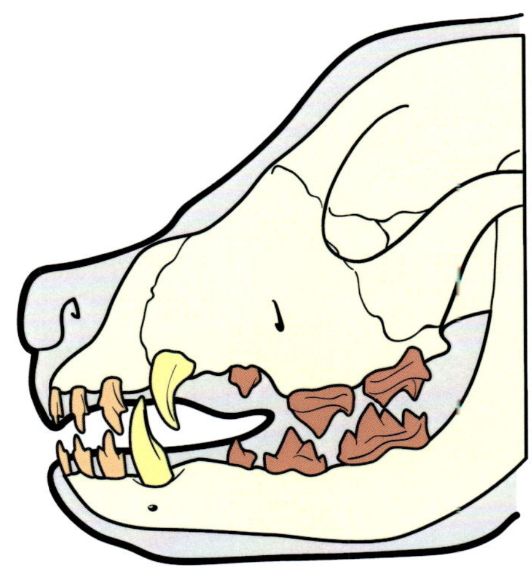

- i: Incisors
- c: Canines
- p: Premolars

4 How many teeth do cats have?

Download a sample odontogram for your use

Cats are strict carnivores and so their teeth differ from those of dogs. However, the soft tissues shown on the sheet are equivalent to those of dogs.

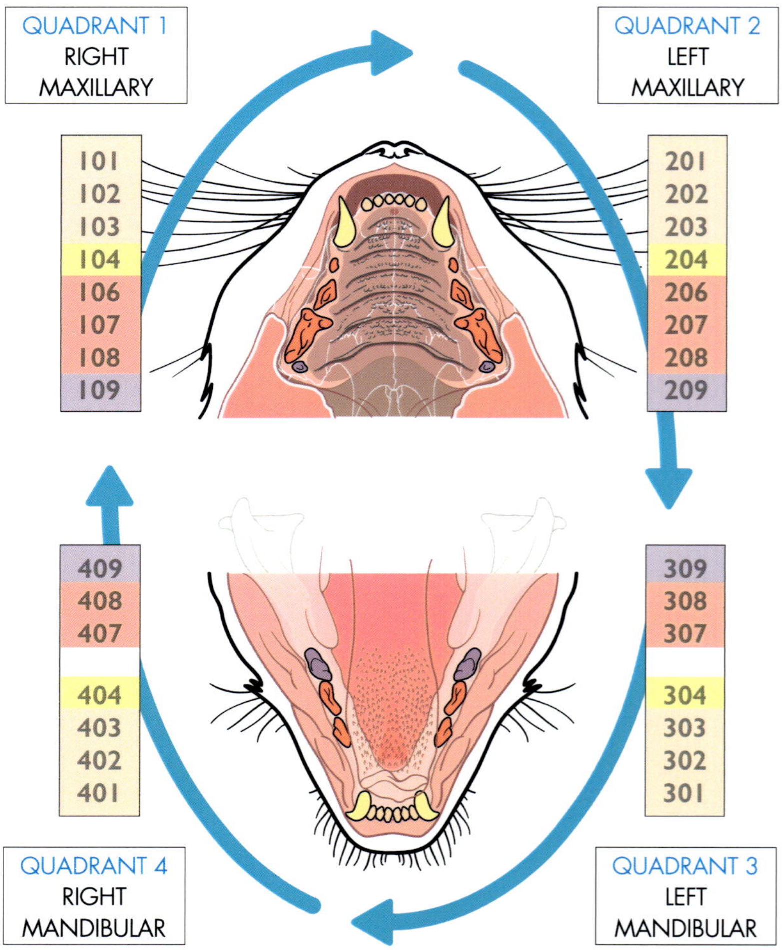

Total dental formula

Kitten

$$2\times\left(i\,\frac{3}{3}\;c\,\frac{1}{1}\;p\,\frac{3}{2}\right) = 26 \text{ teeth}$$

Adult

$$2\times\left(I\,\frac{3}{3}\;C\,\frac{1}{1}\;P\,\frac{3}{2}\;M\,\frac{1}{1}\right) = 30 \text{ teeth}$$

Number of roots	Maxillary teeth	Mandibular teeth
1	I, C, P2	I, C
2	P3, M1	P3, P4, M1
3	P4	—

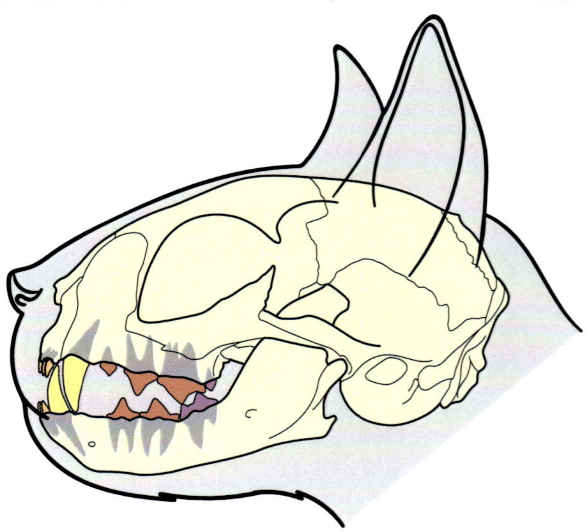

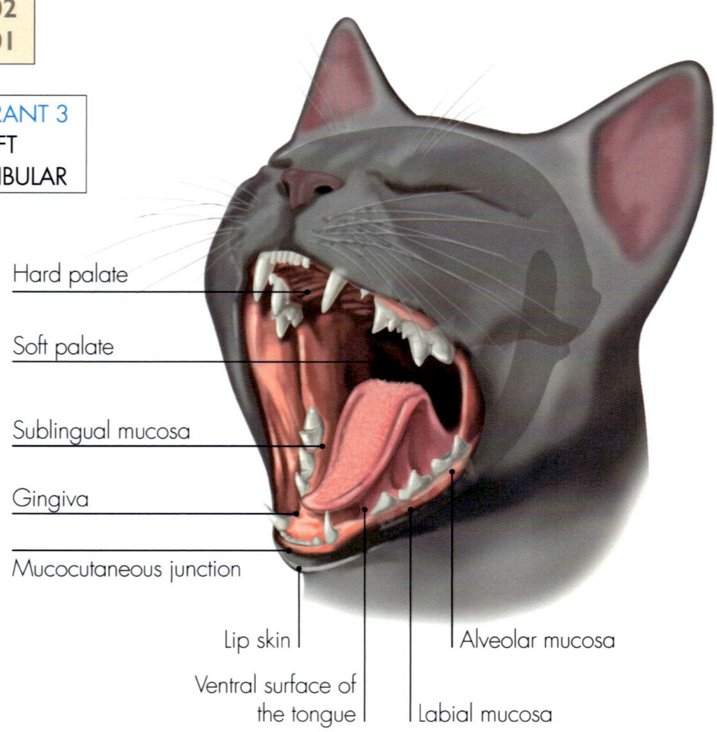

5 Dental eruption

Teeth begin to form during embryonic development, continue to develop after birth, and begin to erupt across the gum surface within a few weeks of birth. Throughout this process, animals present a mixed dentition in which both deciduous and permanent teeth can be seen.

After 6 months of age, any milk teeth that have not yet fallen out should be extracted (see Sheet 22).

Dogs

Eruption of deciduous teeth (days)

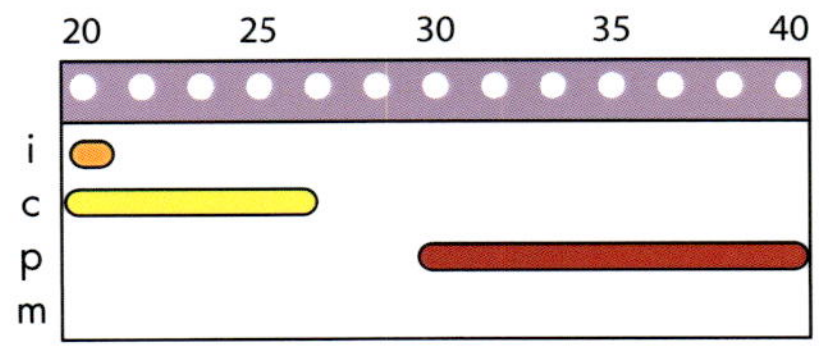

Cats

Eruption of deciduous teeth (weeks)

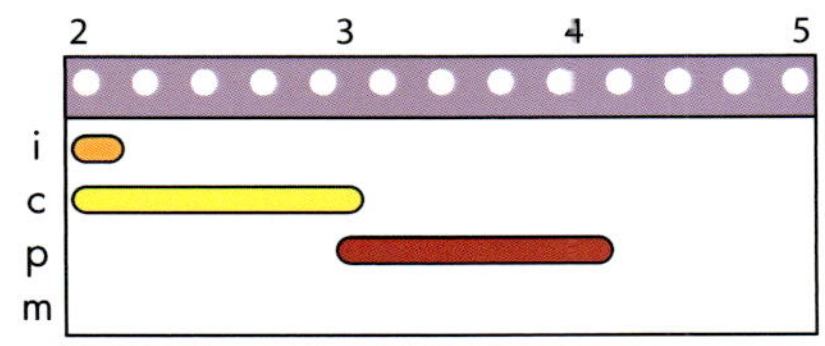

The first teeth to erupt are the central incisors.

Eruption of permanent teeth (months)

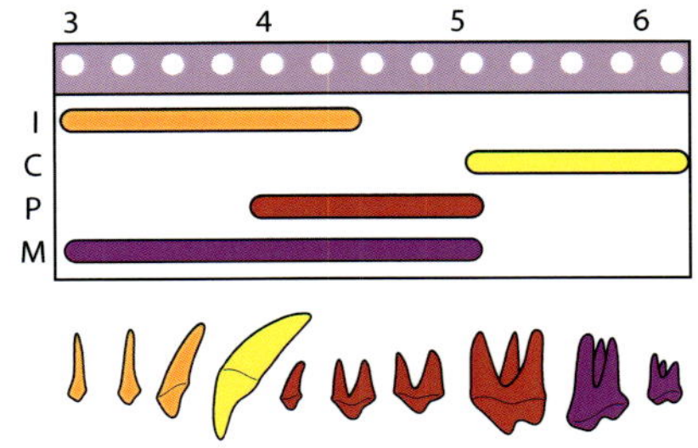

Eruption of permanent teeth (months)

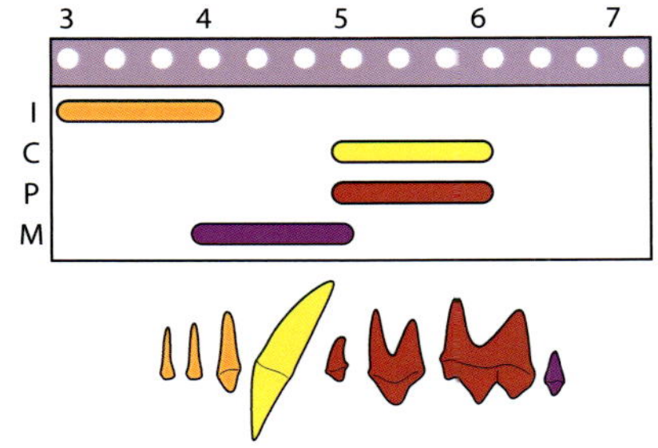

Neither dogs nor cats have deciduous molars.

Tooth eruption

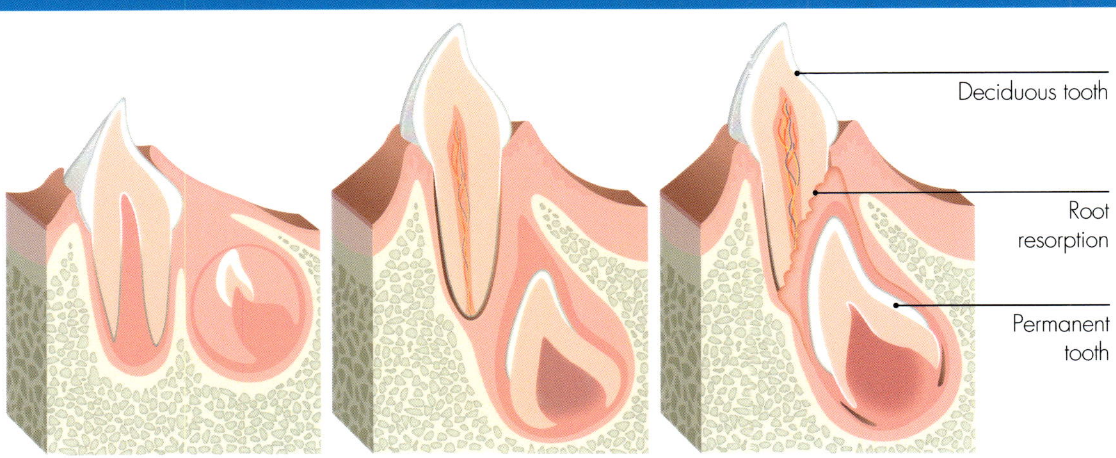

Deciduous tooth eruption

Full development of the deciduous tooth in the bony alveolus

Progressive development of the permanent tooth

6 Tooth and periodontium anatomy

Teeth are anatomical structures comprising tissues of different density and hardness, located in the oral cavity and whose main function is chewing. The periodontium is the anatomical unit that serves to hold the tooth in the bone and suspends it so that it can resist the force of chewing and the normal use of the teeth.

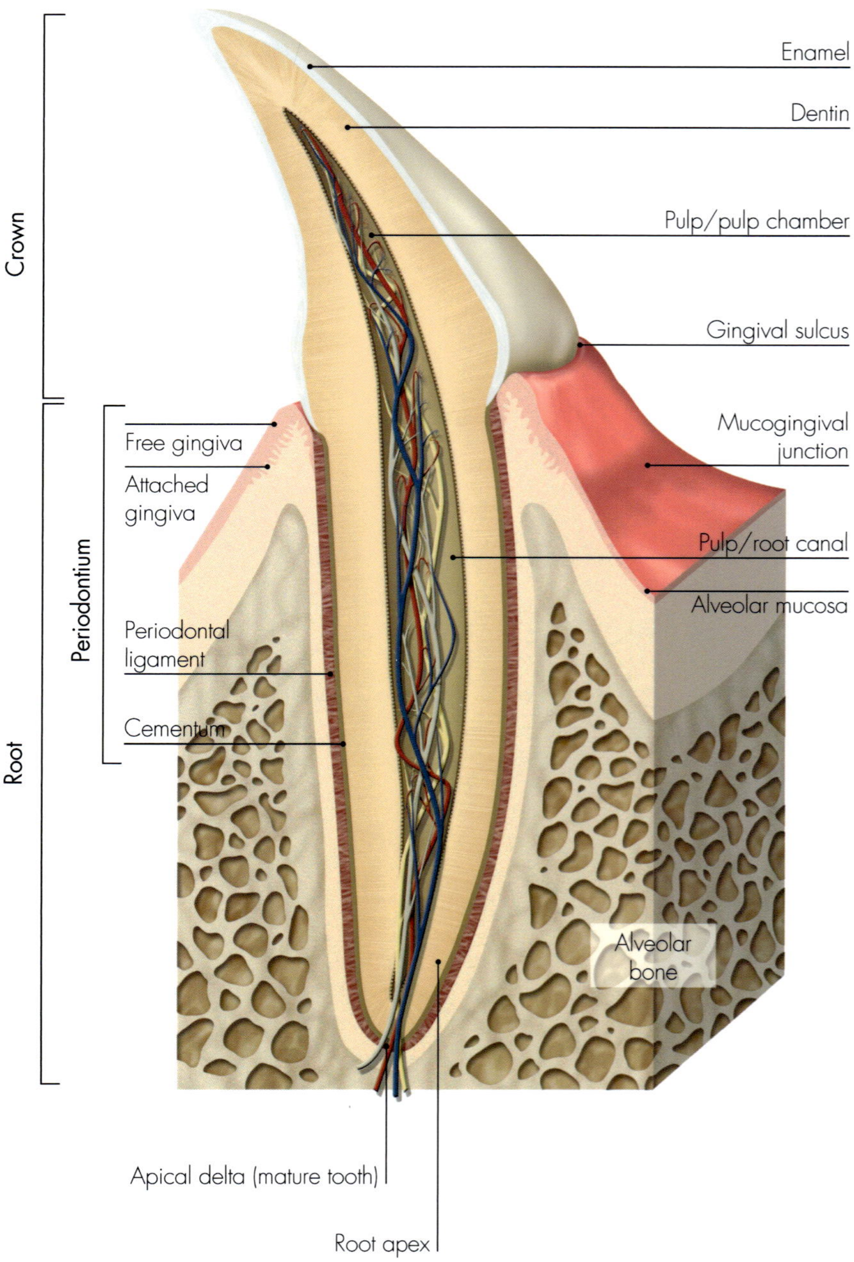

Considerations

In teeth, enamel is the hardest and most mineralized tissue and has no regenerative or reparative capacity. Dentin is less hard than enamel but harder than bone, and it constitutes a major part of teeth and continues to be deposited throughout life (secondary dentin).

The root apex in immature teeth is a single, very wide opening, while in mature teeth it forms the apical delta, with numerous apical openings or branches.

The periodontium is formed by the free gingiva, which forms an invagination between the tooth and the gingiva, called the gingival sulcus (measuring 0.5–3 mm), by the periodontal ligament, which acts as a shock absorber against masticatory forces, and by the avascular and highly mineralized cementum, which itself is involved in repair and resorption processes throughout life.

The alveolar process is the bone that houses the tooth, providing it with nutrition and support.

Progressive reduction of the pulp because of the growth of secondary dentin

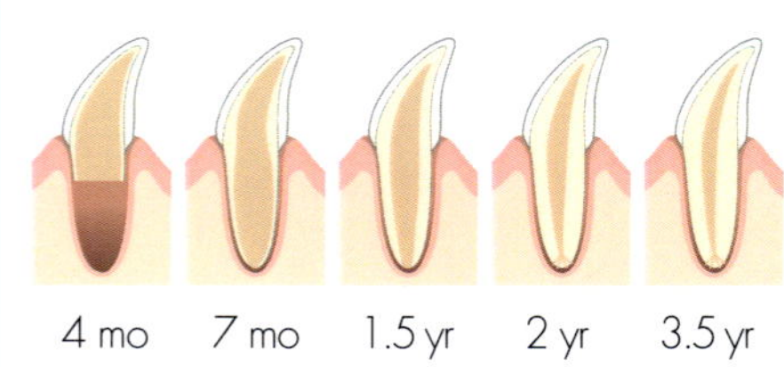

7 Oral examination in the veterinary clinic

Oral examination should form part of every general examination given that 80% of dogs and cats from the age of 3 years require some type of dental treatment. Prevention is fundamental because pets tend not to show pain and only stop eating when the pathology is very advanced.

The information gathered from an oral examination of a conscious animal is limited, and only a preliminary diagnosis can be made. A definitive diagnosis can only be determined under general anesthesia (see Sheet 12).

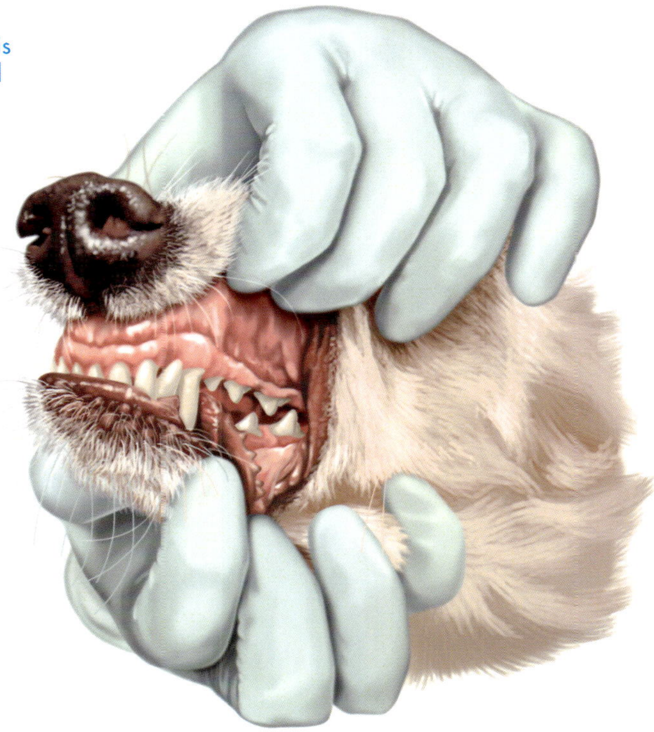

Step 1: Extraoral examination

- Palpation of the bones and muscles of the face: Contact is established with the animal to help them relax. Asymmetries, inflamed/atrophied areas, and painful spots detected by palpation are noted.
- With the mouth closed, the lip is lifted: The buccal and labial aspects of the teeth are observed to check if there is normal occlusion or malocclusion, etc.

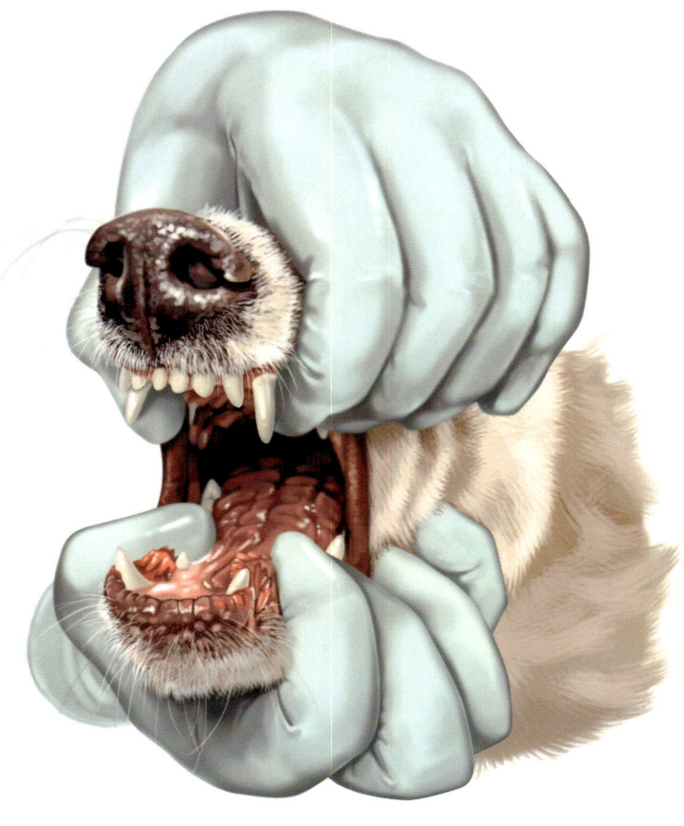

Step 2: Intraoral examination

- **Dogs:** Placing one hand on the muzzle and two fingers behind the canine teeth, the dog relaxes the jaw. Press gently on the mandibular incisors with the other hand.
- **Cats:** Holding the head by the zygomatic arches, gently pull the mancibular incisors downward with the index finger of the other hand.

8 Normal occlusion

Occlusion is the relationship between the teeth of the upper and lower arches. The shape of the head varies in different breeds, so what is considered normal occlusion in one breed may be malocclusion in another. The optimal time to assess occlusion is during an examination of the mouth in the veterinary clinic because the mouth must be closed and must not be impeded by an endotracheal tube.

Conformation of the head

- **Dolichocephalic**: Elongated head.
- **Mesocephalic**: "Middle-sized" head. The description of normal occlusion is based on the conformation of a mesocephalic skull.
- **Brachycephalic**: Short head.

Lateral view

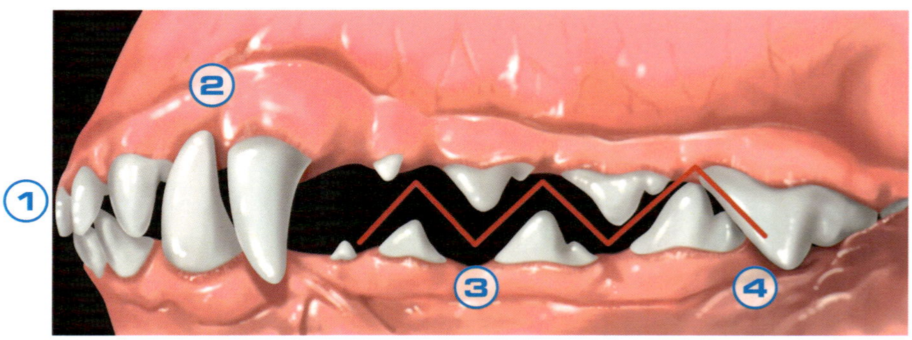

Rostral view

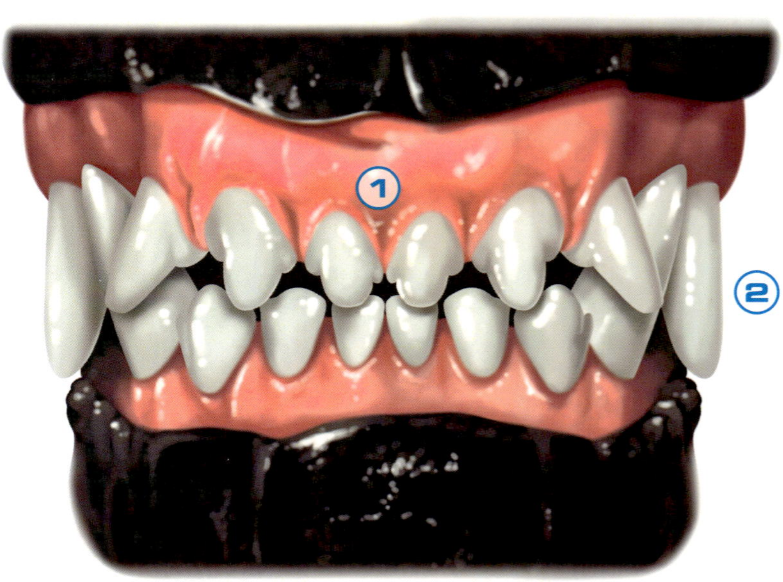

1. Relationship between incisors: Scissor bite. The upper incisors are positioned labially to the lower incisors.
2. Canine occlusion: The mandibular canine is situated equidistant in the space between the maxillary canine and the third incisor.
3. Relationship between premolars: Zigzag interdigitation; the cusps of the premolars occlude with the interdental spaces of the opposing arch without contact between them.
4. Carnassial teeth: The maxillary fourth premolar occludes with the buccal aspect of the mandibular first molar; this achieves a powerful cutting effect.

Clinical significance

Dogs should have functional and comfortable occlusion:

- They should not damage the gums or mucosa with their own teeth when chewing.
- No excessive wear (or fractures) should be present due to contact between the teeth.

9 Dental malocclusion

The term malocclusion refers to abnormal positioning of the teeth. Class I malocclusion or dental malocclusion is defined as one or more misplaced teeth, regardless of whether there is a discrepancy between the length or width of the facial bones. In general, this type of malocclusion is not considered hereditary.

Early detection

Any malocclusion can produce trauma to tissues or other teeth when the dog (or cat) closes the mouth, but animals do not show the pain produced by these lesions and so they are rarely detected by owners. If not treated in time, complications are frequent, including oronasal communication, abrasions, and dental fractures. Malocclusion can also be accompanied by behavioral changes such as hyperactivity or destruction of items, which come to an end when malocclusion is resolved. Therefore, this disorder should be detected at an early age, during the animal's first visits to the veterinarian.

Lingualization of the mandibular canines

- This is the main cause of dental malocclusion.
- It occurs when the mandibular canine teeth erupt toward the tongue (linguoversion). When closing the mouth, the canine teeth contact the palatal mucosa instead of reaching the diastema between the maxillary canine and third incisor.

Lingualization of the mandibular canine teeth requires treatment because it is extremely painful, even if dogs do not show pain. If this problem is not detected in time, the palate can become perforated, producing an oronasal communication.

Lingualization. Rostral view

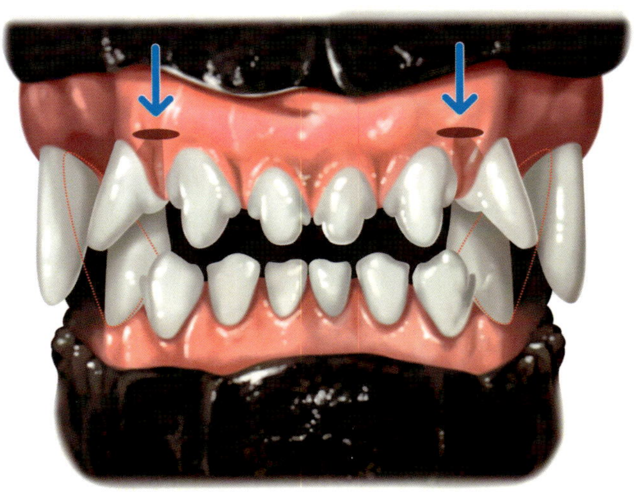

Palatal view

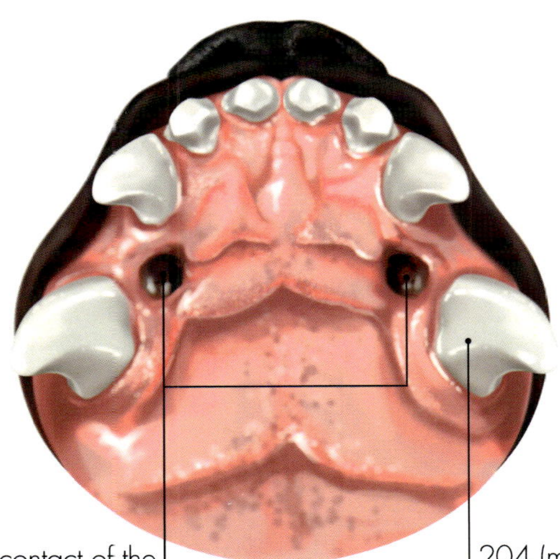

Treatment options for malocclusion

1. Extraction of the teeth causing occlusal trauma (see Sheet 39).
2. Crown reduction and subsequent pulp treatment (see Sheet 43).
3. Orthodontic correction (see Sheet 44).

10 Skeletal malocclusion

Skeletal malocclusion occurs when there is a discrepancy between the width and/or length of the maxilla and that of the mandible. In general, this type of malocclusion is considered to be hereditary.

Class II malocclusion: Mandibular distocclusion or brachygnathism

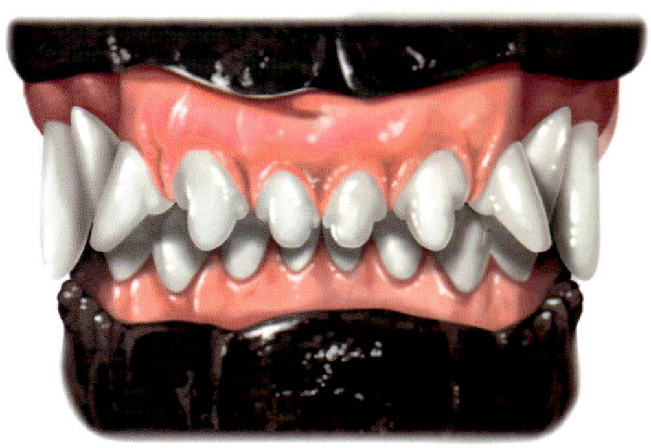

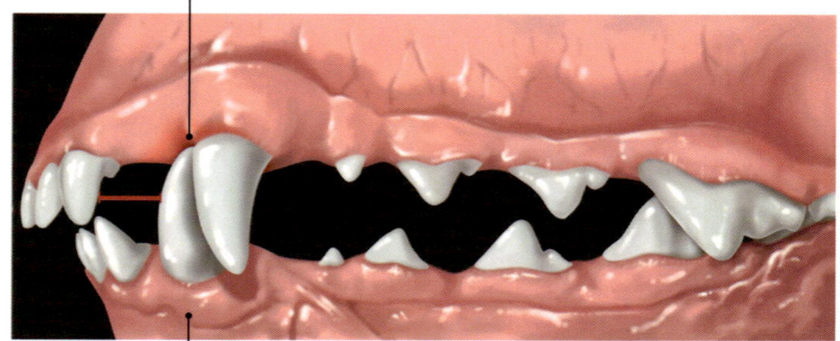

Class III malocclusion: Mandibular mesiocclusion or prognathism

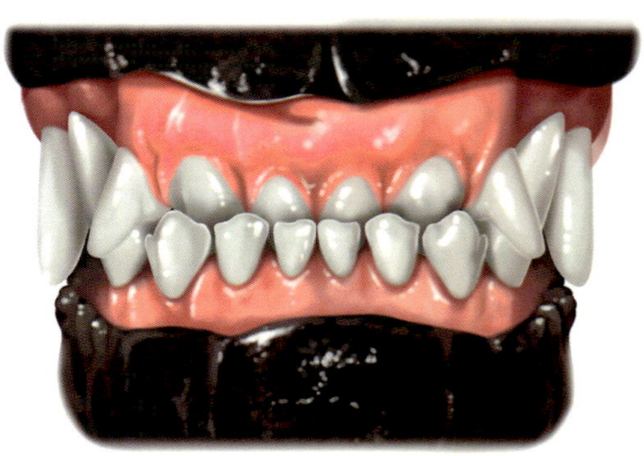

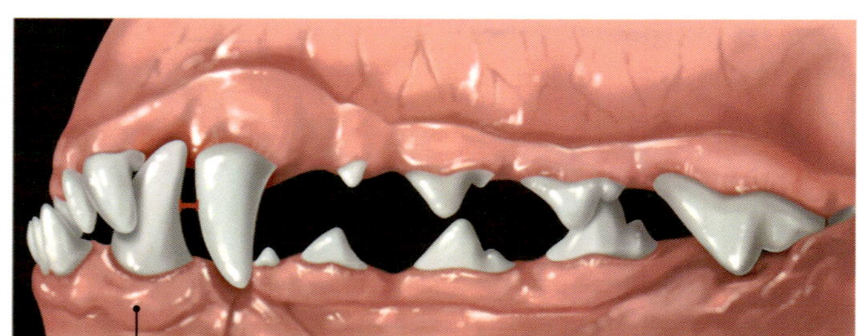

Treatment

If damage to soft tissues or other teeth occurs when closing the mouth, treatment is required, even if the animal shows no signs of pain.

Purely aesthetic malocclusions do not require treatment, and most veterinary associations worldwide advise against it for ethical reasons.

11 Malocclusion in cats

Both skeletal and dental malocclusion problems are also found in cats. Cats of brachycephalic breeds are more prone to suffer from this disorder because of the shape of their jaw, which is shorter and wider than in other breeds.

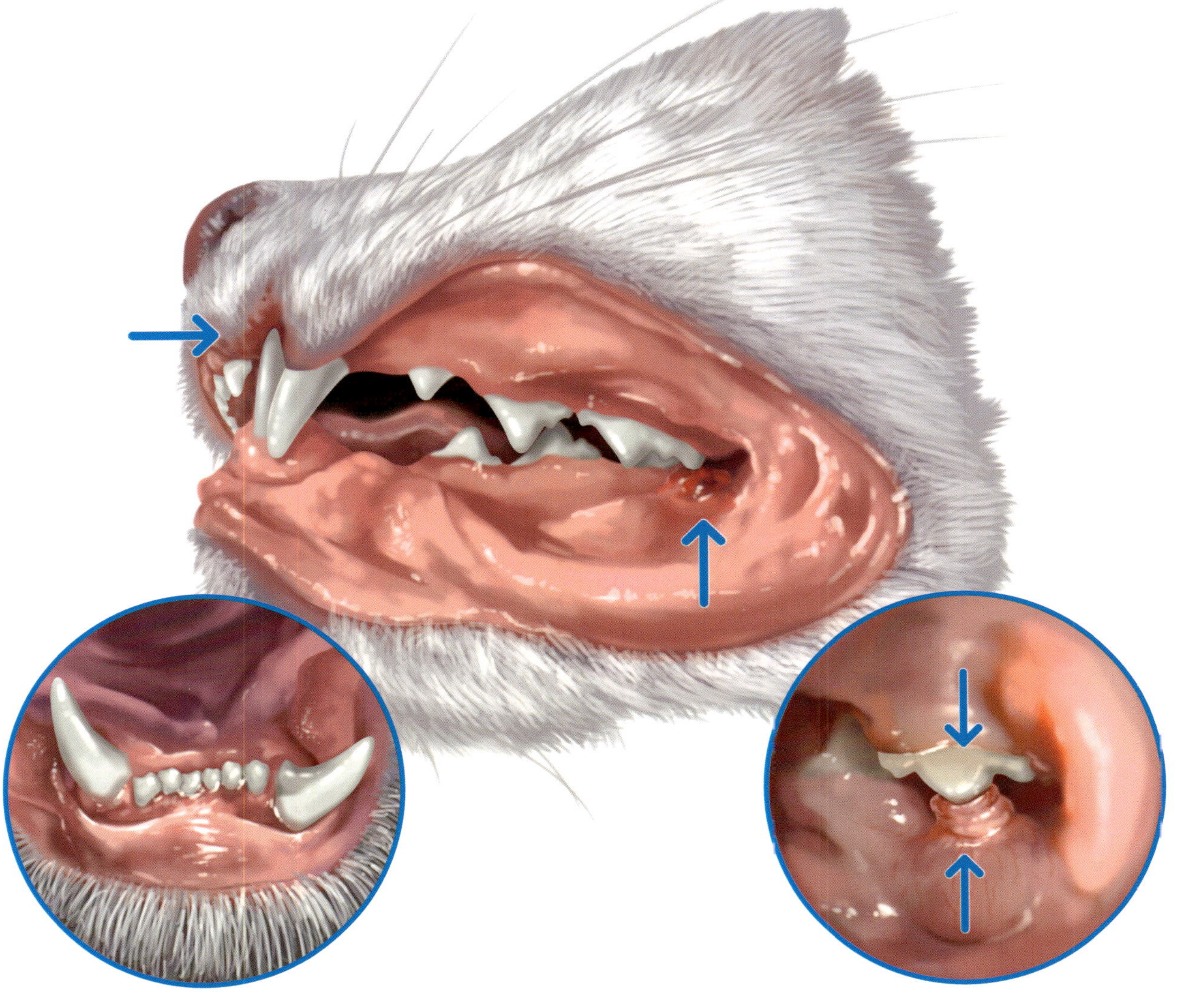

The deviated mandibular canine causes injury to the lip by continued contact

Continuous traumatic contact between the maxillary fourth premolar and the mucosa of the mandibular first molar often results in inflammatory proliferation or pyogenic granuloma

Treatment

- If malocclusion is exclusively an aesthetic problem, no treatment is necessary.
- If the alteration in the tooth position produces contact between the teeth or damage to the tissues, orthodontic treatment is required (see Sheet 44), which will have to be performed by a specialist in veterinary dentistry.
- Odontoplasty is used to reduce the size of the crown of the tooth causing the trauma. Modification of the crown requires root canal therapy (partial or total pulpectomy) and restoration (see Sheet 43).
- Extraction of the malocclusive tooth/teeth may also be necessary (see Sheet 39).

12 Oral examination under general anesthesia

Any surgical procedure in the oral cavity must be performed under general anesthesia with endotracheal intubation in order to:

- Adjust the type of anesthesia administered to each patient (appropriate ventilation and monitoring).
- Protect the respiratory tract to avoid the risk of aspiration of debris, blood, calculus, and the water used to cool the dental handpieces.
- Provide pain management. Most dental procedures are painful and require adequate analgesia.

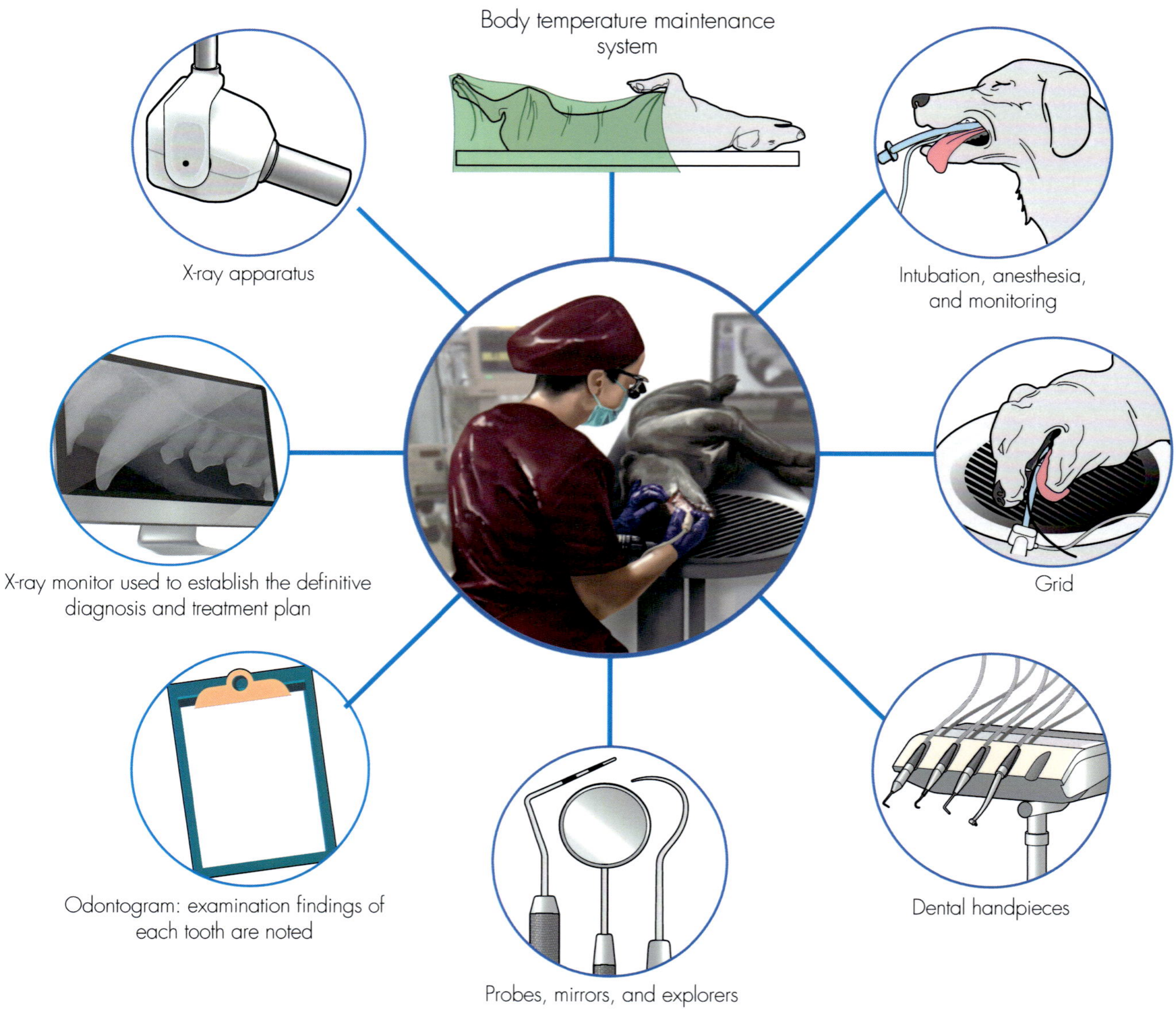

The World Small Animal Veterinary Association (WSAVA), as well as the European and American Veterinary Dental Colleges (EVDC and AVDC), strongly advise against performing dental procedures without anesthesia. Sedation as a means of restraint is also not recommended because it jeopardizes the quality of the treatment the patient receives and poses a high risk of aspiration.

13 Intraoral radiography: Importance and techniques

Indications

- Clinical signs of periodontal disease.
- Prior to tooth extraction, to confirm the need for extraction and plan the appropriate technique.
- After tooth extraction, to avoid leaving root remnants and check that the bone was not damaged during the procedure.
- After any change in tooth color (pulp pathology).
- Dental defects: Fractures, cavities, wear and tear, resorptive lesions.
- Oral neoplasms, to assess bone involvement.
- Maxillofacial trauma.
- Diagnosis of missing teeth.

Materials

- Radiographic film or digital sensors.
- X-ray emitters. Dental X-ray emitters allow radiographs to be taken without moving the patient, facilitating the procedure
- Image display systems.

Intraoral radiography is essential in all dental treatments. General anesthesia is required.

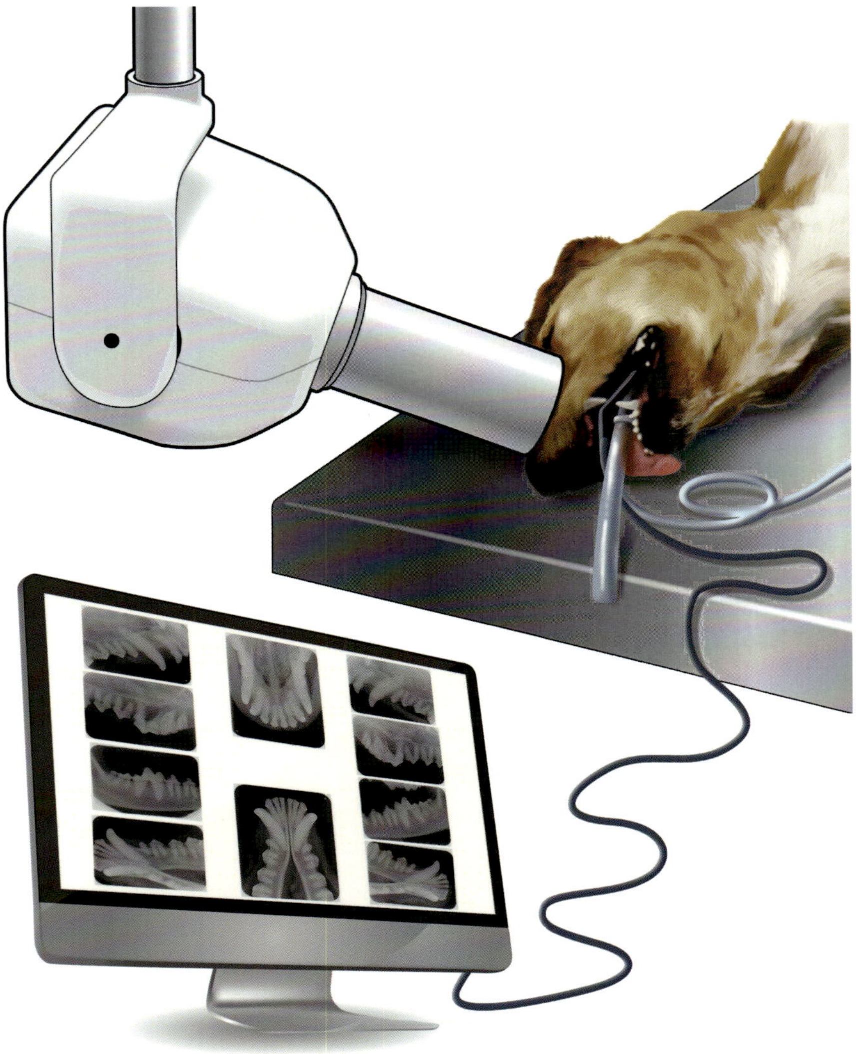

Paralleling technique

For mandibular premolars and molars

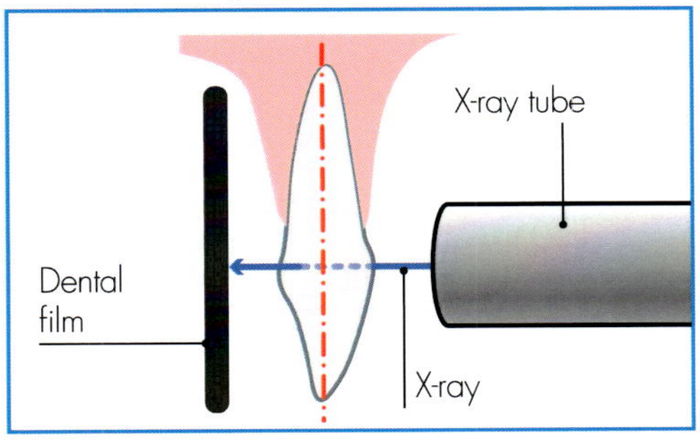

Bisecting technique

For all the other teeth

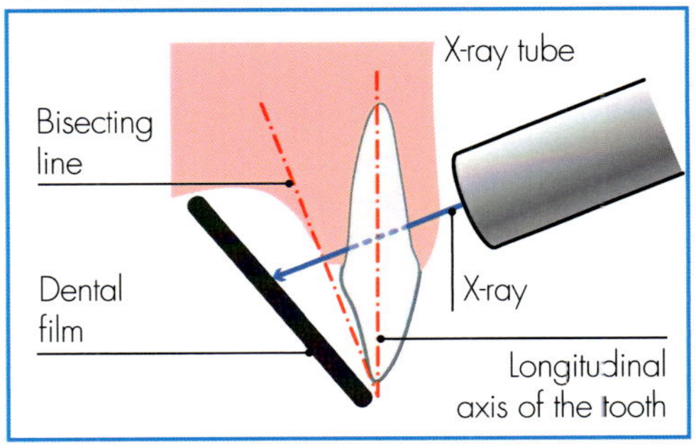

14 Typical scenario: 2–3-year-old dog

Periodontal disease is the most common disorder in companion animals, with more than 80% of dogs aged over 2 years suffering from this problem. This is an inflammatory disease of the periodontal tissues in response to plaque bacteria.

Gingivitis and periodontitis are the two expressions of periodontal disease.

Gingivitis—inflammation of the gums—is the earliest sign of the disease and is reversible.
If the bacterial plaque is eliminated by brushing, gingivitis will disappear and gum health will be restored.

Bacterial plaque
A soft, sticky layer on the tooth surface comprising bacteria and food debris. It can be easily removed by daily tooth brushing (see Sheets 19 and 20). Bacterial plaque present for more than 48 hours causes gum inflammation.

Gingivitis
The accumulation of bacterial plaque on the teeth causes inflammation of the gums.

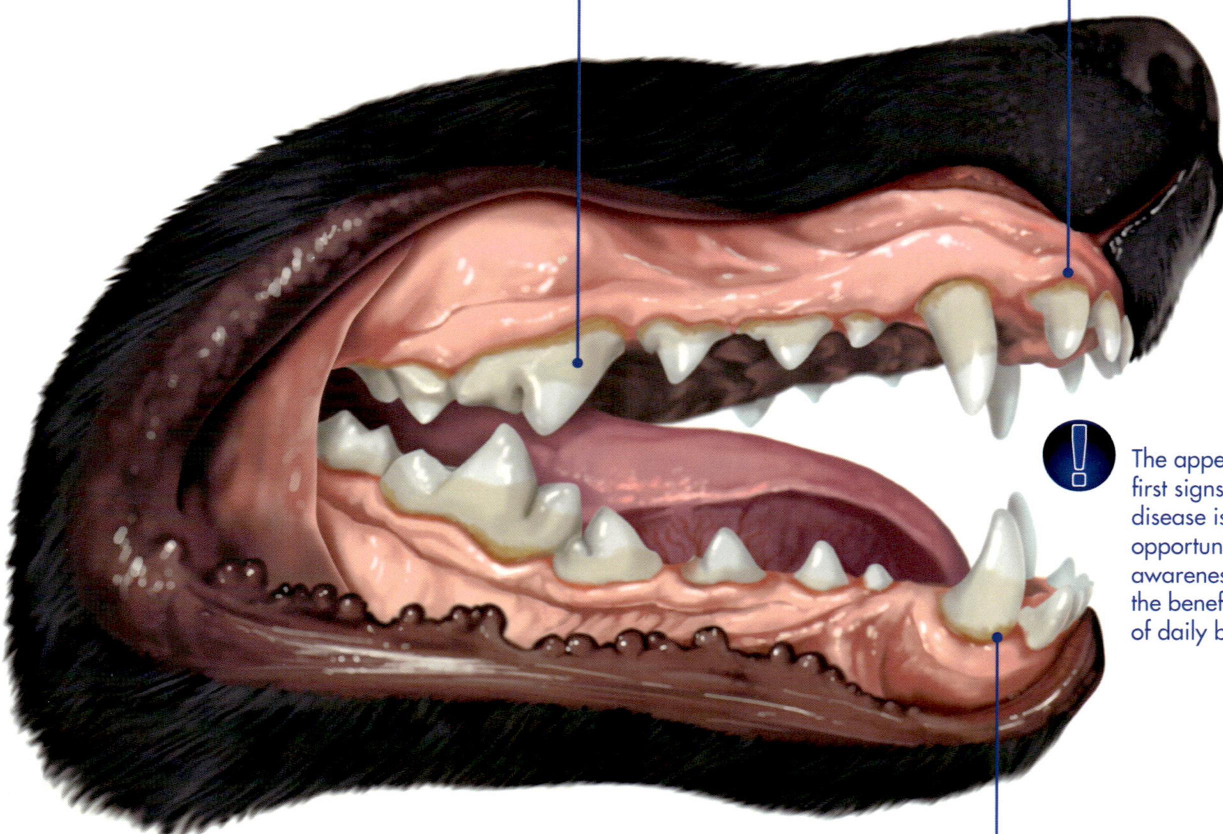

The appearance of the first signs of periodontal disease is a good opportunity to raise the awareness of owners of the benefits to their pets of daily brushing.

Both gingivitis and periodontitis can be observed even before one year of age in animals predisposed to periodontal disease. The ages indicated on the sheet titles are purely indicative.

Calculus or tartar
Bacterial plaque and mineral salts in the saliva and crevicular groove mineralize and form calculus or tartar. This is a side effect of poor hygiene. It is not pathogenic, but its irregular surface favors the accumulation of even more bacterial plaque.

Professional dental cleaning

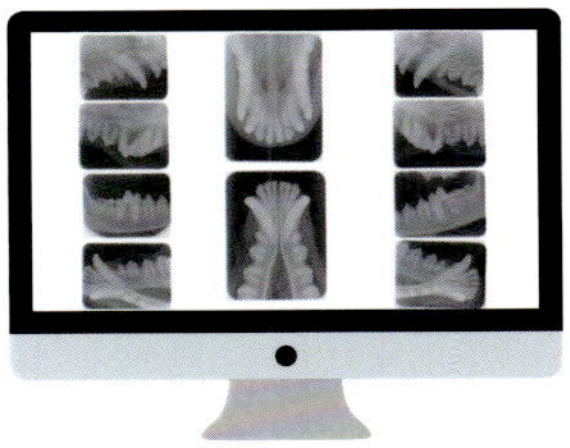

To avoid periodontitis, professional—both supragingival and subgingival—dental cleaning must be performed under general anesthesia.

Supragingival cleaning

This is performed by ultrasound, with subsequent polishing of the enamel, to remove visible calculus from the surface of the teeth. A low-power setting should be used at a 45° inclination, with abundant irrigation with water and for only a few seconds on each tooth. This is to avoid producing thermal or mechanical damage that could compromise tooth vitality (which is very painful for the patient). With the elimination of tartar and subsequent polishing, the smooth surface of the enamel is restored and the daily elimination of bacterial plaque by brushing is facilitated (see Sheets 19 and 20). Oral chlorhexidine is the safest and most effective antiseptic against bacteria in the mouth, and when used just before professional periodontal treatment, it reduces the bacterial load of the aerosol generated by ultrasonic devices. For postoperative plaque control, the owner can administer oral chlorhexidine every 12 hours for 1–2 weeks.

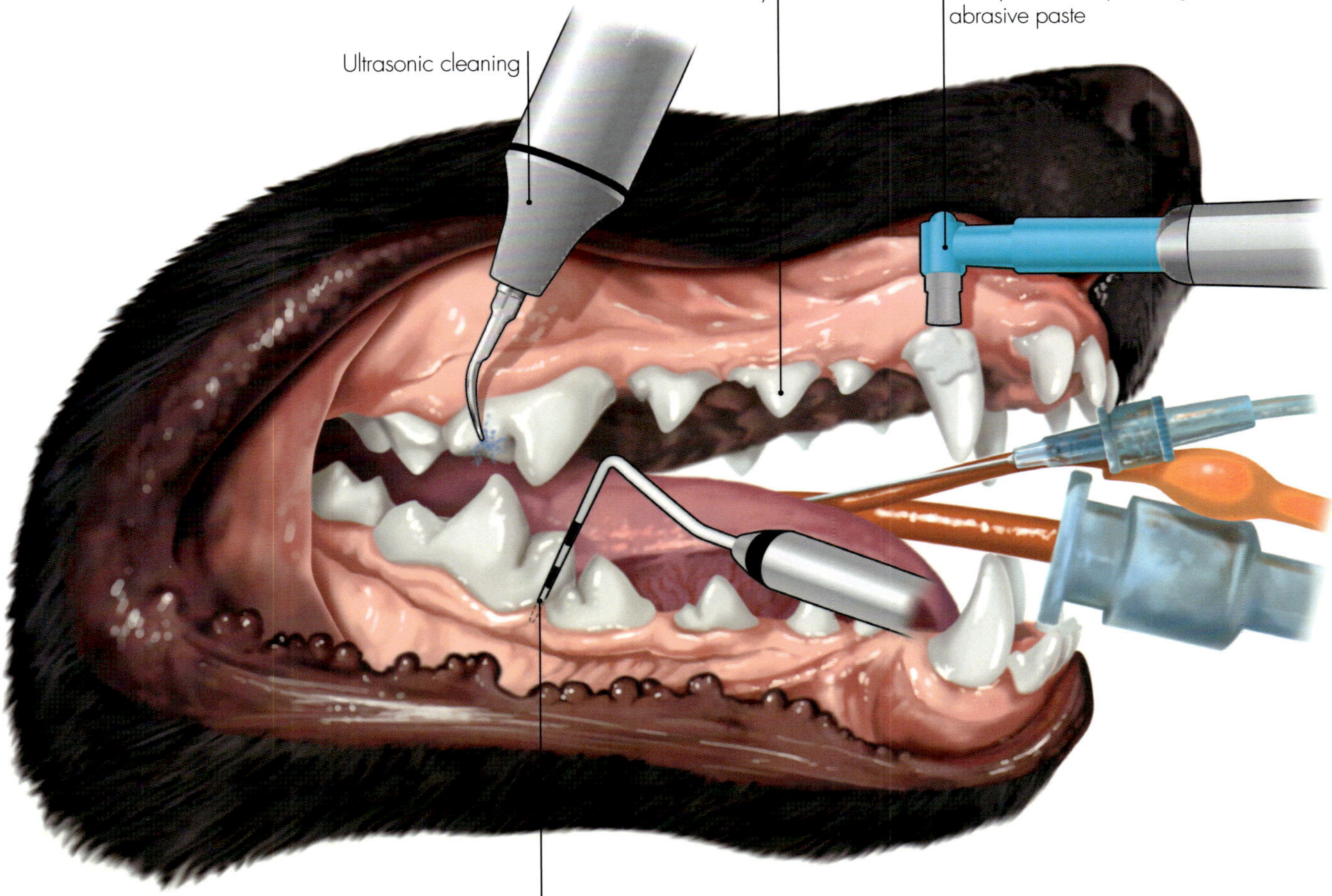

Subgingival cleaning

This removes invisible calculus (under the gums) and is the most important part of the treatment because it prevents progression to periodontitis (loss of the supporting structures of the tooth). This type of cleaning requires specialized training in the use of both periodontal inserts and manual curettage instruments for subgingival cleaning.

No dental procedures should be performed under sedation. See the recommendations of the World Small Animal Veterinary Association (WSAVA).

15 Typical scenario: 3–5-year-old dog

Without proper treatment and brushing of the teeth, periodontal disease progresses, and destruction of the tooth support, bone loss, and gingival recession begin to occur, leading to periodontitis.

The progression of the disease depends on the immune response and genetic predisposition of the animal. In some breeds the progression is faster and the onset earlier. For example, greyhounds and small-sized breeds are more predisposed to periodontitis. In contrast, other dogs may not develop periodontitis despite a high accumulation of plaque and calculus or tartar.

Increased accumulation of visible calculus (tartar) and hidden lesions
Calculus builds up due to the constant presence of bacterial plaque. Even so, increased calculus is not indicative of the severity of the disease because most lesions are hidden. Thus, cleaning the visible calculus is insufficient to control the disease, and untreated hidden lesions perpetuate infection and discomfort.

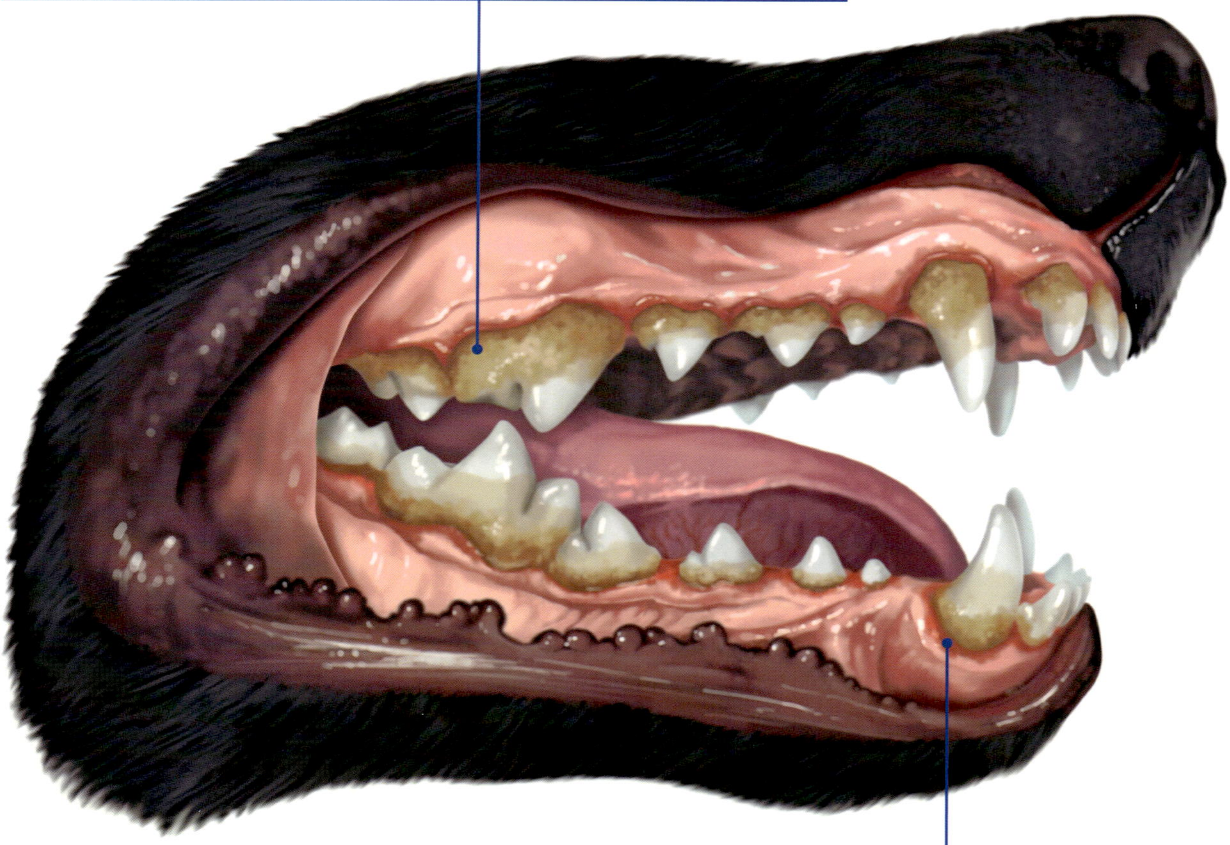

Gingivitis
Swollen and reddened gums that bleed easily.

Increased severity
When gingivitis persists over time, tooth junctional epithelium destruction begins and a periodontal pocket forms in which even more plaque can accumulate. If inflammation persists without treatment, bone resorption begins.

The goal of treatment is to maintain clinically healthy gingivae in order to prevent disease progression. General anesthesia, intraoral radiography, and periodontal probing are required. Without a diagnosis, cleaning only has aesthetic value.

Progression

Untreated gingivitis can progress to periodontitis. In this case, the inflammation progresses, producing gum recession, loss of tooth support, and the formation of periodontal pockets. One or more teeth may be affected, and each tooth should be diagnosed and treated accordingly because incomplete treatments favor the progression of the disease.

All the findings for each tooth are noted on an odontogram to evaluate the evolution of the patient at their next visit.

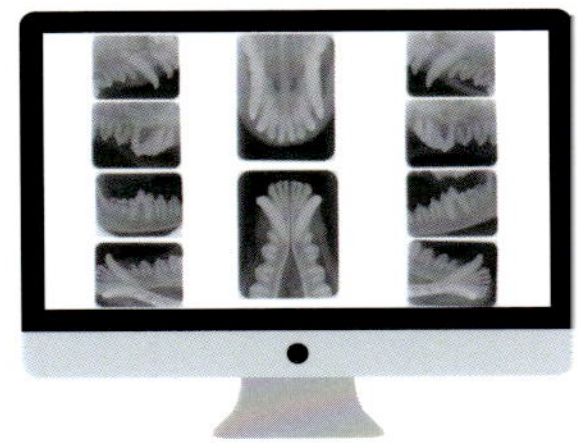

Intraoral radiography, together with the examination and periodontal probing findings, is essential to determine the true extent of bone loss.

Gingival recession and root exposure
When bone loss occurs, the gingiva irreversibly recedes. Exposed roots require advanced periodontal treatment (scaling and smoothing) to prevent the accumulation of bacterial plaque. This treatment stops the progression of periodontal disease, but maintenance via daily brushing by the owner remains essential.

Furcation defects
This is the loss of bone at the root trunk of teeth with two or more roots. Without daily brushing, the bone at the furcation will continue to be destroyed, even more rapidly than in other areas.

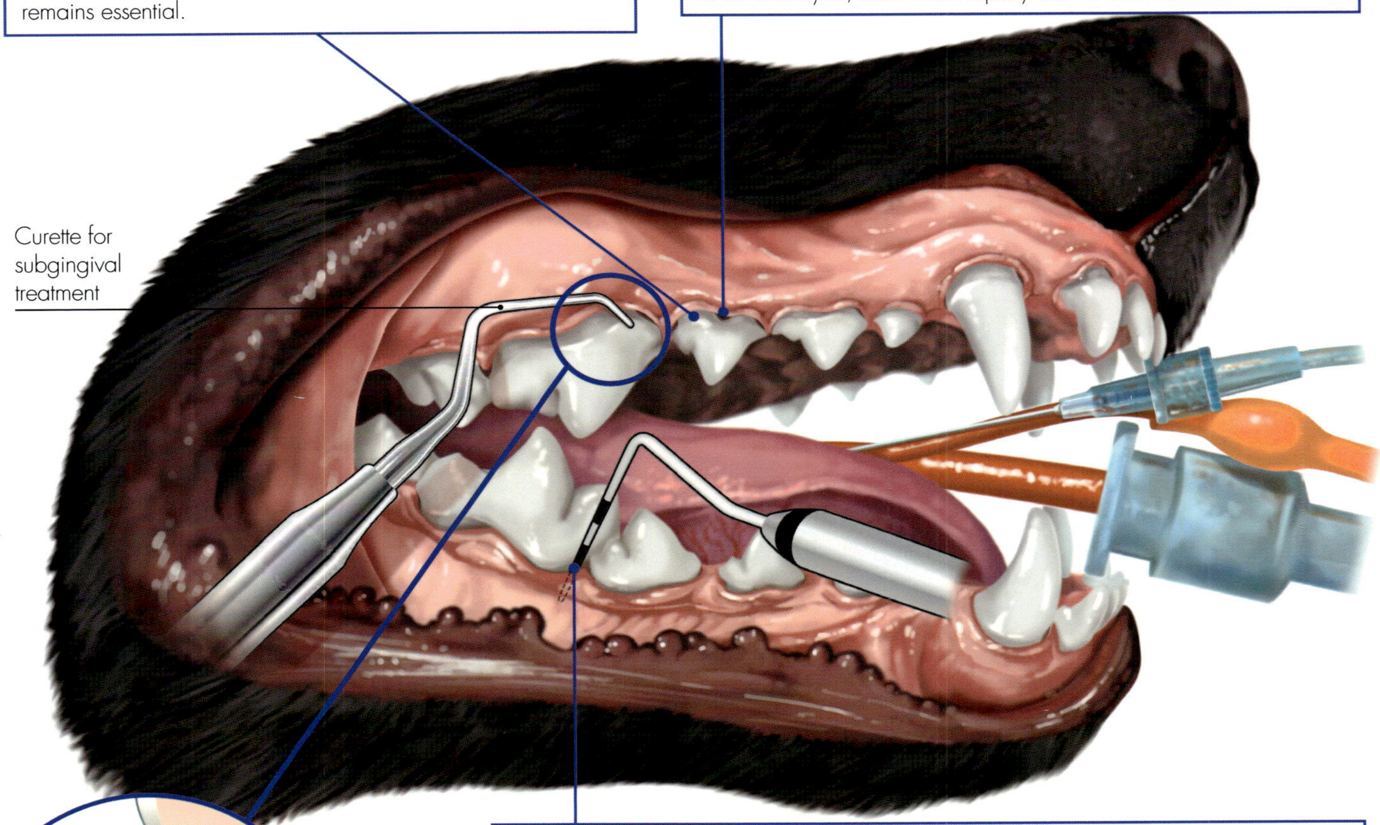

Periodontal probing
This technique is used to measure the depth of any periodontal pockets and invisible bone loss. Deep periodontal pockets (>5 mm) require tooth extraction or advanced periodontal treatments (see Sheets 39 and 40). Provided the owner is able to perform good daily brushing, these treatments help to eliminate infection of the deep pockets and can even partly regenerate the supporting tissues of the tooth.

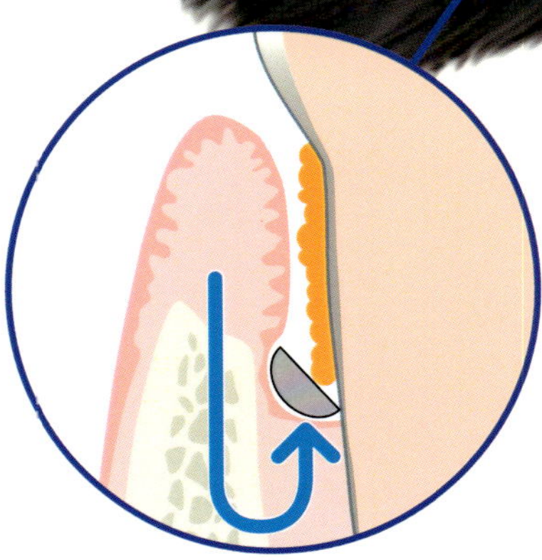

4 mm periodontal pocket
Subgingival curettage is required: Subgingival debridement and root planing.

16 Typical scenario: 5–7-year-old dog

Animals with advanced periodontitis show no signs of discomfort, so most owners delay having their pet undergo any periodontal treatment. A common concern is that pets will not be able to eat without their teeth, but in fact it is just the opposite: it is much harder for them to eat with tooth pain. After the necessary treatment and extractions, animals usually regain vitality, their appetite improves, and they play like when they were younger. Veterinarians play a fundamental role in conveying information to owners about the local and systemic consequences of periodontitis on the health of their pet (see Sheets 17 and 18) as well as the need for complete periodontal treatment (see Sheet 40).

Increased accumulation of calculus (tartar) is not indicative of the degree of periodontitis because calculus is the mineralization of bacterial plaque on the tooth surface and is not inherently pathogenic.

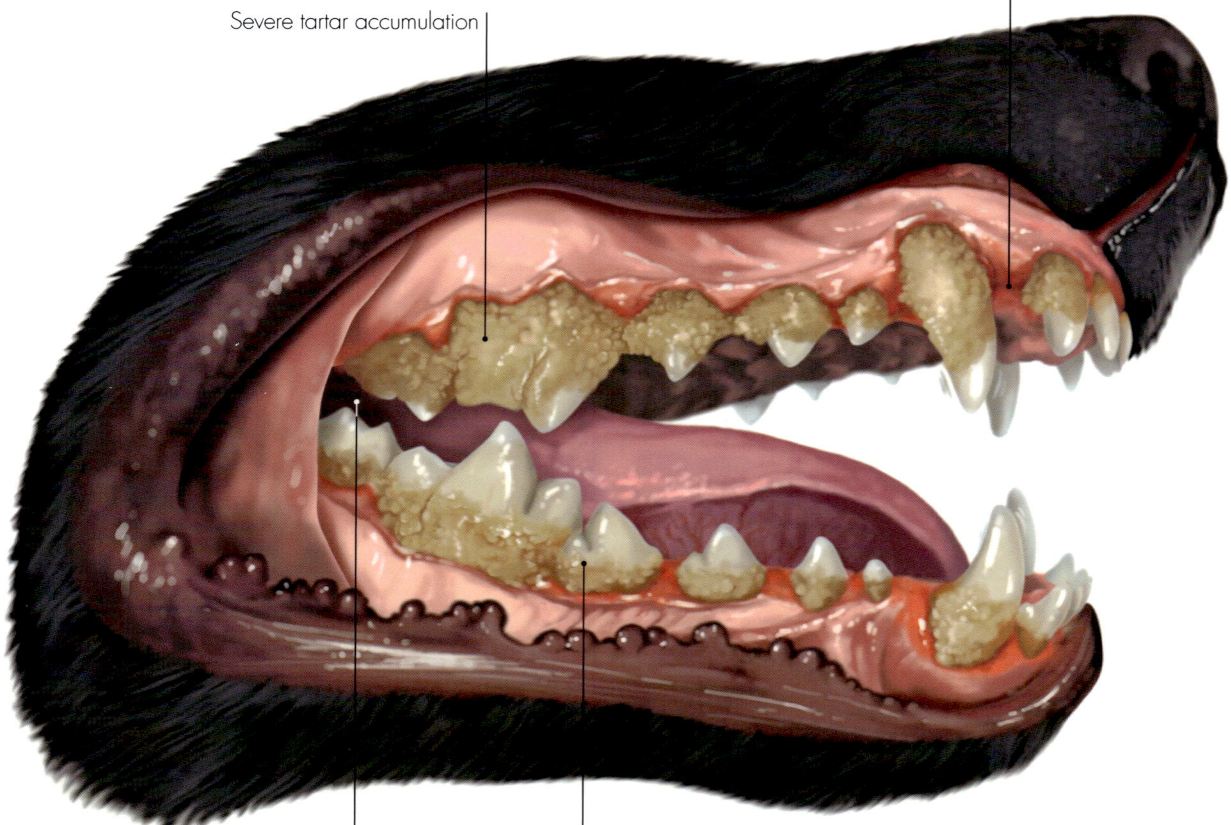

The true extent of the disease is hidden beneath the gums and must be assessed individually for each tooth by oral examination under general anesthesia, periodontal probing, and intraoral radiography.

Systemic antibiotics are not effective in the control of periodontal disease, and so their use should be reserved for specific cases.

Radiological findings show severe periodontal involvement, requiring multiple tooth extractions.

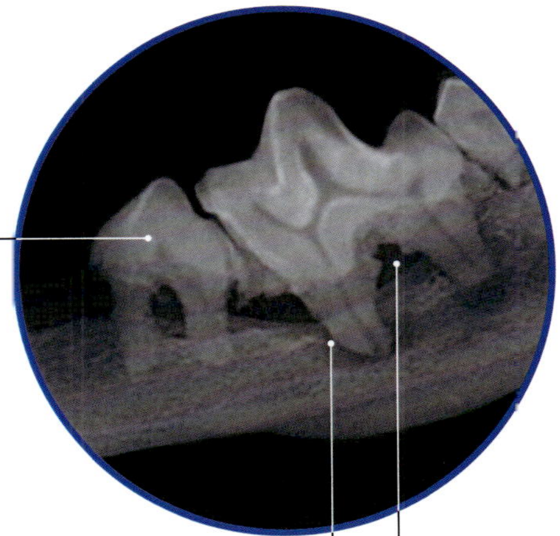

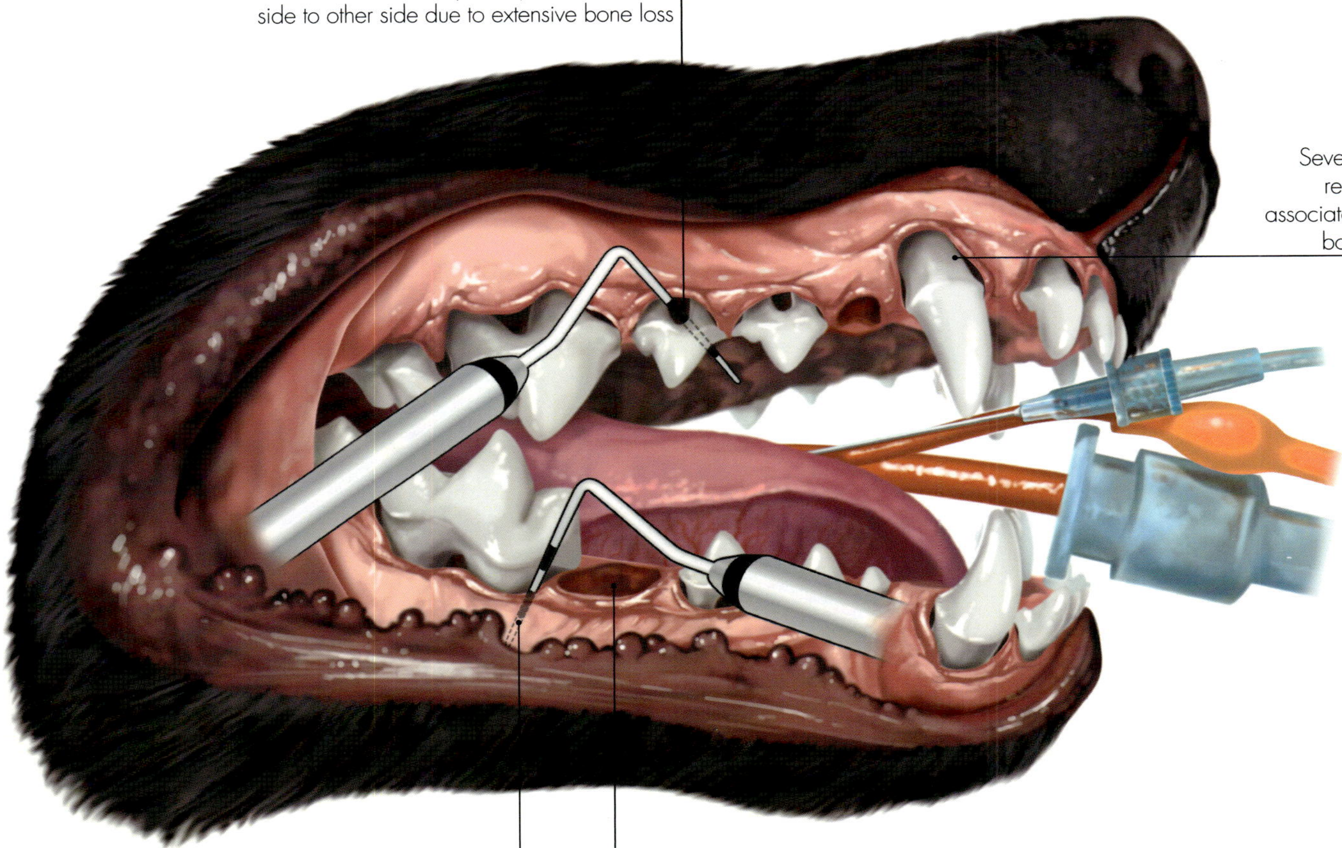

Periodontal treatments should not be performed in conjunction with other "clean" surgical procedures under the same general anesthesia.

Treatment

Extraction of any mobile teeth, with more than 25% of support loss and deep periodontal pockets, that cannot be preserved by advanced periodontal techniques.

17 Local sequelae

The true extent of periodontal disease and associated bone destruction is often underestimated until severe external signs appear. A thorough examination under general anesthesia and intraoral radiography prior to any oral treatment avoids these complications.

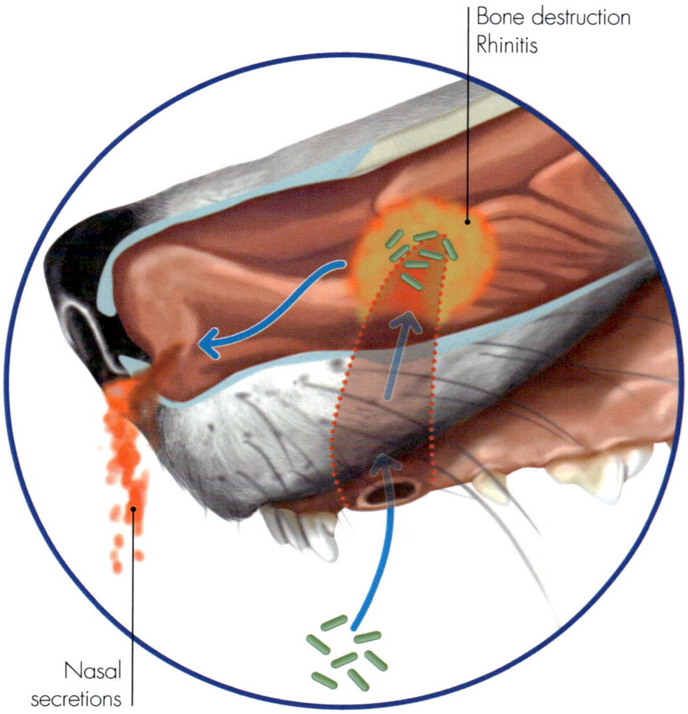

Oronasal communication and fistula

Destruction of the bone separating the tooth from the nasal cavity may not be apparent until an examination is performed under general anesthesia with periodontal probing and intraoral radiography (see Sheet 13).

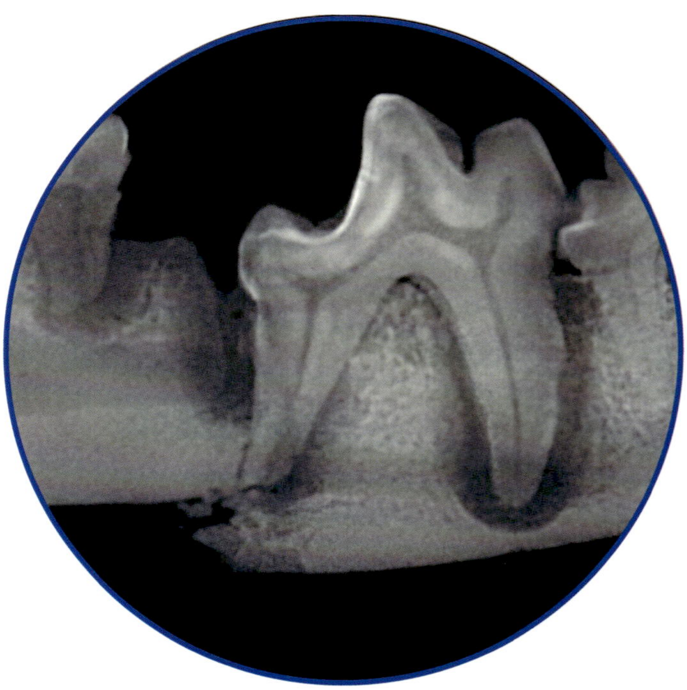

Pathological fractures

Small-sized breeds have larger teeth relative to their skull size compared to larger breeds. Therefore, the horizontal and vertical bone loss that occurs in cases of chronic periodontitis poses a high risk of mandibular fracture in these breeds.

Fracture of the weakened bone may occur during dental extraction or even in everyday situations such as getting off the couch or playing.

18 Systemic sequelae

The destruction of periodontal tissues and the bone surrounding the tooth can have serious effects on the health of the animal. Deep periodontal pockets provide a favorable anaerobic environment for bacteria to multiply, and these bacteria can enter the bloodstream causing damage to organs such as the heart, liver, or kidneys.

The main problem with periodontal disease is that it is hidden beneath the gums, and so it is too often underestimated because the disease is not externally visible. Superficial tartar cleaning does not eliminate the infection and creates a false sense of security in the owner of having done the right thing while the animal continues to suffer from the effects of chronic infection.

Animals with chronic periodontitis have a diminished quality of life.

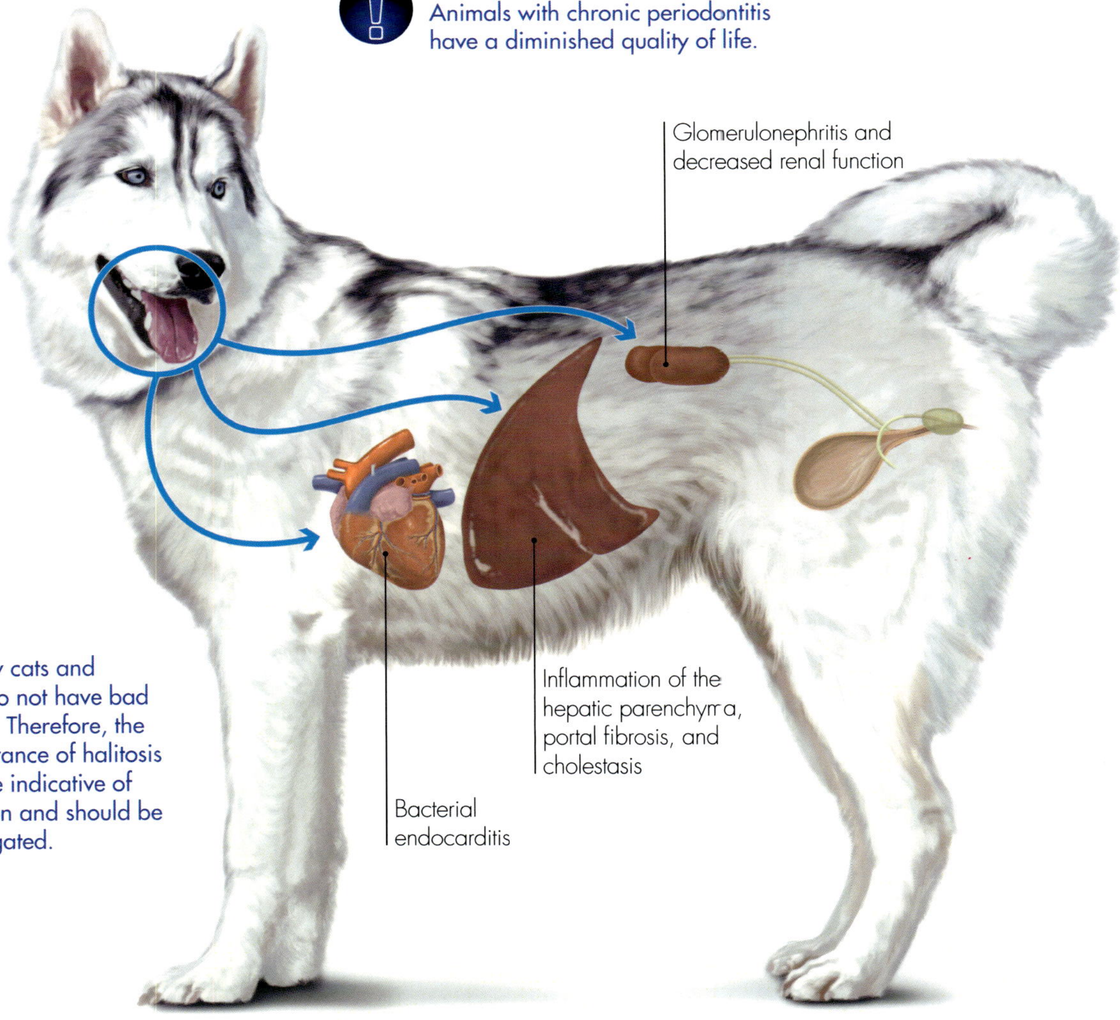

Healthy cats and dogs do not have bad breath. Therefore, the appearance of halitosis may be indicative of infection and should be investigated.

Antibiotics

Due to the complex organization of bacteria in this disease, antibiotic therapy fails and should not be used routinely or as a substitute for appropriate periodontal treatment.

Diabetes

Diabetic patients are predisposed to suffer from severe periodontitis, which in turn generates further insulin resistance. This is why these animals require regular periodontal treatment.

19 How to brush a dog's teeth

Daily tooth brushing is the best clinically proven method to remove plaque, prevent the onset of periodontal disease, and ensure the health of our pets.

Closed mouth and raised lip: The lingual and palatal aspects of the teeth accumulate less plaque (the tongue contributes to their cleaning) but do also need brushing
When the dog is used to the procedure, open their mouth to also brush these surfaces

There are brushes especially designed for pets, but brushes for people (soft or medium hardness) are also suitable
Angle the brush at 45° so that the bristles penetrate the gingival margin

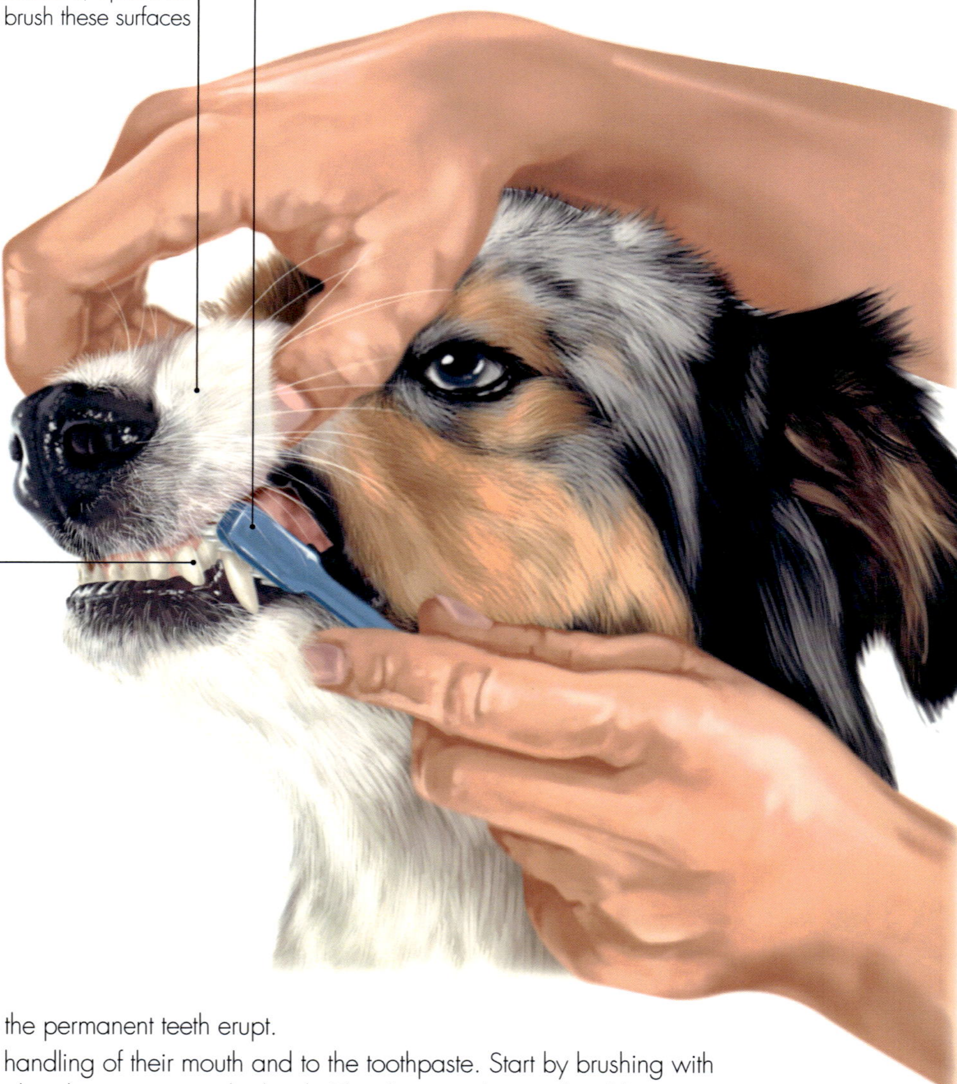

Never use toothpaste for people; if ingested by pets, it produces gastric irritation and the taste is not suitable for them. The pastes formulated for dogs are highly palatable and can serve as a positive stimulus for brushing (and so it is worth finding the one that the dog likes the most).

The visible teeth on both sides are brushed with up-and-down or circular movements in this order: canines, premolars, molars, and incisors
The incisor area is highly sensitive, so dogs tend to reject manipulation in that region

Tips

1. **Start at an early age:** Even before the permanent teeth erupt.
2. **Go slowly:** Get the animal used to handling of their mouth and to the toothpaste. Start by brushing with gauze and when the dog is used to this, then start using the brush. The dog must be comfortable!
3. **Establish a daily routine:** The habit benefits both the pet and the owner.
   Tooth brushing can be added on to any other preestablished routine.
4. **Use positive reinforcement:** Use toothpaste with a pleasant taste and reward the dog after brushing with a toy or a walk.
5. **There are always exceptions:** Do not start accustoming a pet to brushing if there is already pathology and pain, as the dog will likely reject handling. Dogs with aggressive or violent tendencies may require prior training and therapy before brushing will be accepted (consult a veterinarian specialized in behavior).

20 How to brush a cat's teeth

Tooth brushing in adult cats can be somewhat more complicated than in the case of dogs, although it all depends on our commitment and the cat's character. It is much easier to introduce a brushing routine when the cat is still a kitten.

The success of brushing depends on the motivation of the owner, cooperation of the pet, use of the proper technique, and advice given by the veterinarian and assistant/nurse. The effort made by everyone involved will be rewarded by the enormous benefits in terms of improving the pet's health.

Once a day for less than 1 minute will be highly beneficial!

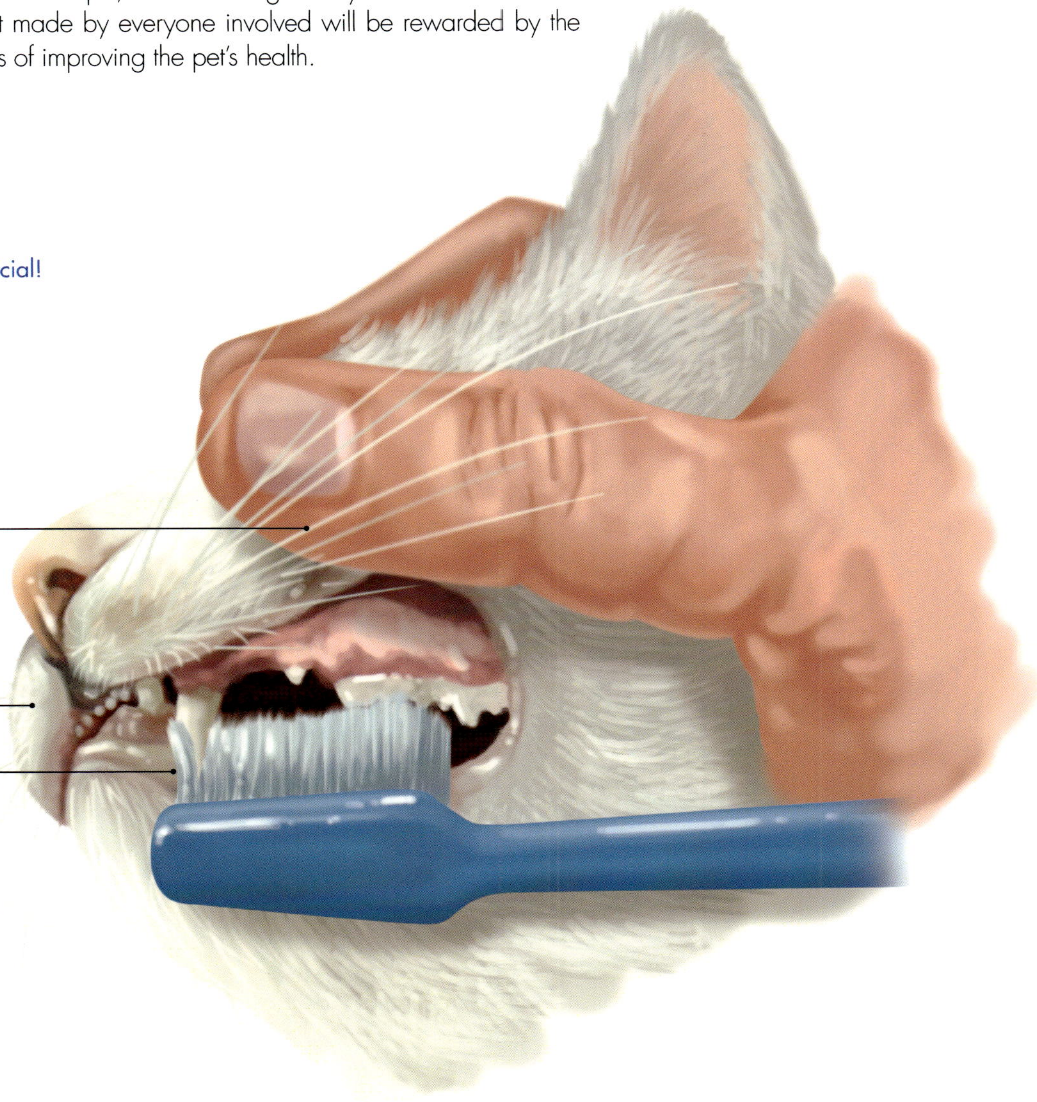

Tips

1. Start by massaging the gums with your finger so that the cat gets used to you handling their mouth.
2. Offer the cat the toothpaste to check if they like it. If the cat does not like it, look for another flavor or do not use any toothpaste at all. Brushing alone, or with water, is still effective.
3. In the first few days, use gauze or cloth wrapped around your finger. When the cat is used to handling, start using a small, soft toothbrush, which is more effective.
4. Brush the areas that accumulate more bacterial plaque first (premolars and molars).
5. If the cat does not want to cooperate, do not force them. It is always better to stop and resume brushing at a calmer time. Once the routine is established, brushing all the teeth can be completed very quickly.

21 Tooth brushing accessories and extras

Numerous studies have demonstrated the efficacy of specific dental diets and dental chews or sticks in reducing the accumulation of calculus and bacterial plaque. Because of the wide variety of products on the market, it is advisable to consult with your veterinarian to choose products with proven efficacy through clinical studies.

Nonetheless, daily tooth brushing remains the most effective method to prevent the progression of periodontal disease, and there is no magic pill that allows us to avoid brushing teeth (both in ourselves and our pets). However, the use of some of these products helps to reduce the accumulation of plaque and tartar and is a helpful addition to daily brushing. Even so, they do not maintain clinically healthy gums in the absence of daily brushing.

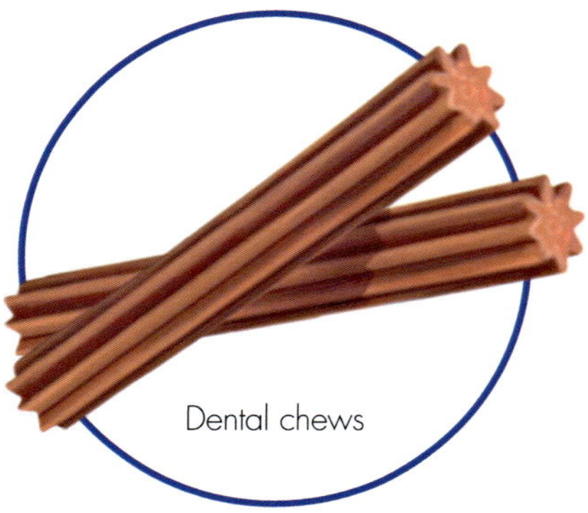

Dental chews and diets
These have been specifically designed to reduce bacterial plaque and calculus buildup in cats and dogs. Some products contain enzymes and substances that prevent or delay the accumulation of plaque and calculus (chemical effect), while others have a texture that helps clean the teeth and a size that increases the chewing time (mechanical effect).

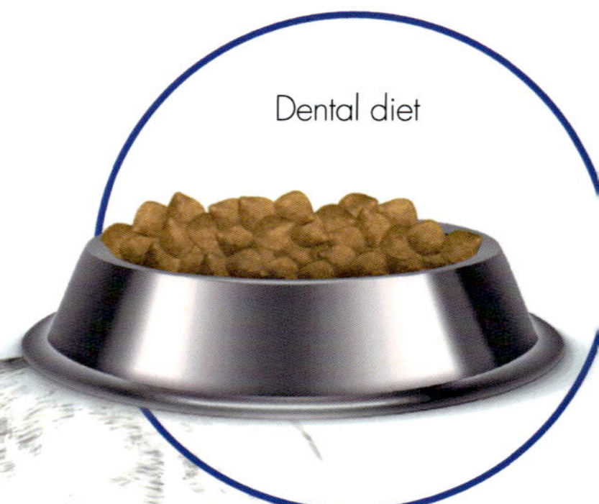

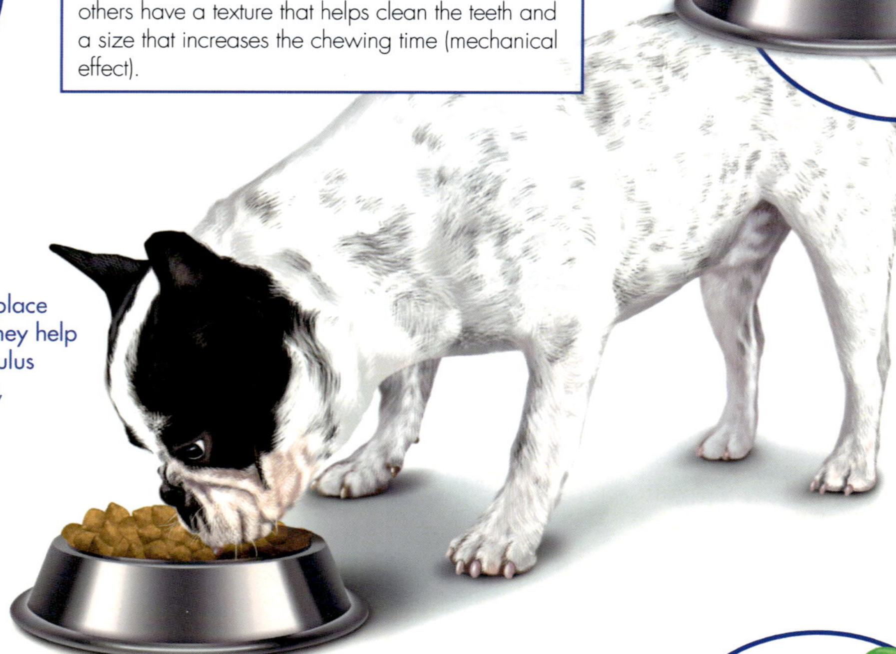

None of these products replace daily tooth brushing, but they help to reduce plaque and calculus buildup and, consequently, the degree of gingivitis.

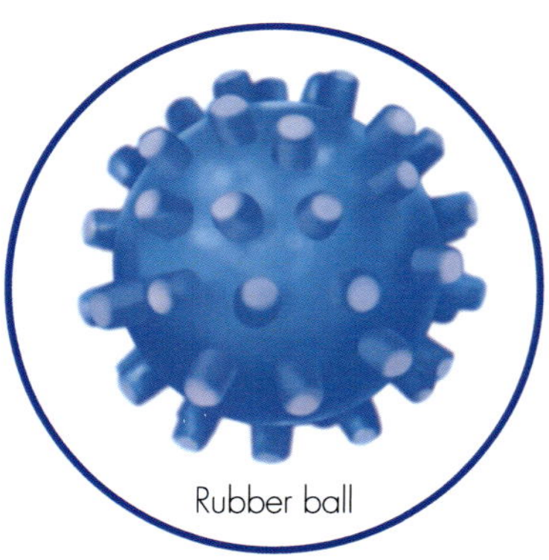

Toys
These should be of a moderate hardness to avoid dental fractures and of a size appropriate to the size of the cat or dog.

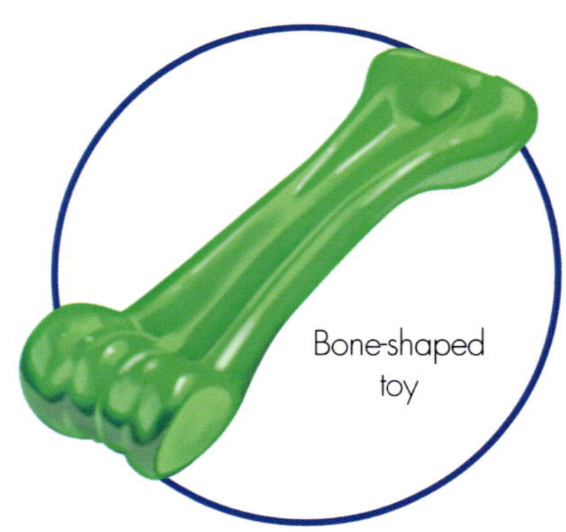

22 Persistent deciduous teeth

Exfoliation of deciduous teeth is often delayed, more commonly in canines and incisors. Small-sized dog breeds are most often affected, with this problem occurring much less frequently in cats.

Extraction?

The deciduous or milk tooth that persists in the mouth once the homologous permanent tooth has erupted should be extracted to avoid displacement of the permanent tooth, malocclusion problems, and the early onset of periodontal disease.

In these cases, intraoral radiography helps to assess whether the permanent tooth has not yet erupted or is absent.

If the permanent tooth is absent and the radiograph shows that the deciduous tooth is healthy, extraction is not necessary, but it should be monitored radiographically on a regular basis because deciduous teeth are more fragile and tend to resorb.

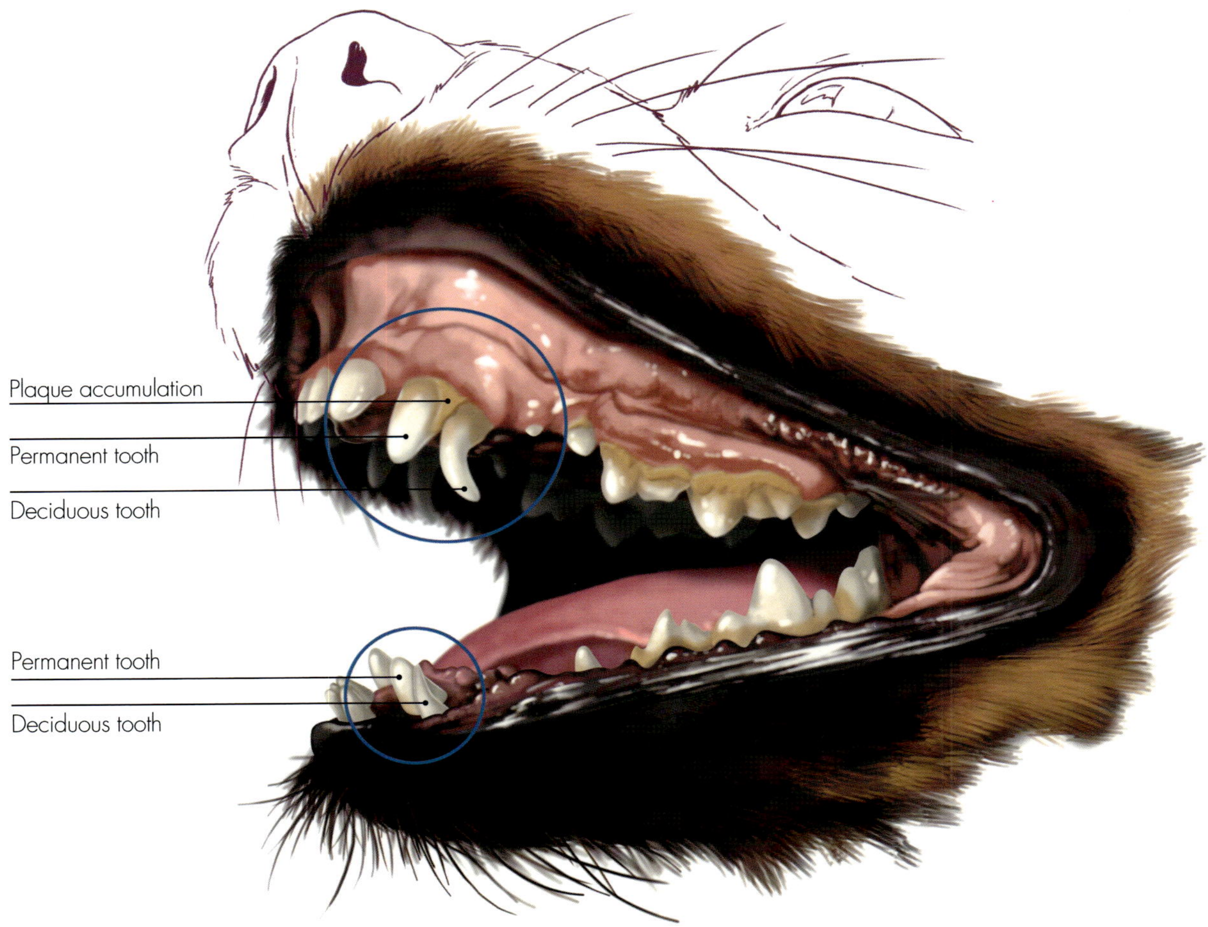

Complications

A common complication is fracture or breakage of milk teeth during extraction. In these cases, the root remnant should be visualized by radiography and extracted using open surgery (see Sheet 39) because it can lead to infection or displacement of the permanent tooth.

Do not wait for persistent decidous teeth to fall out on their own! A milk tooth that persists for more than a few days after the corresponding permanent tooth has erupted should be extracted.

23 Unerupted teeth: Dentigerous cysts

There can be multiple reasons for failure of a tooth to erupt, including genetic factors or developmental diseases. Dentigerous cysts are very common and are associated with unerupted teeth. If a missing tooth is detected in the first few weeks after exfoliation of a deciduous tooth, radiography should be used to confirm if the permanent tooth is truly missing or has not been able to erupt.

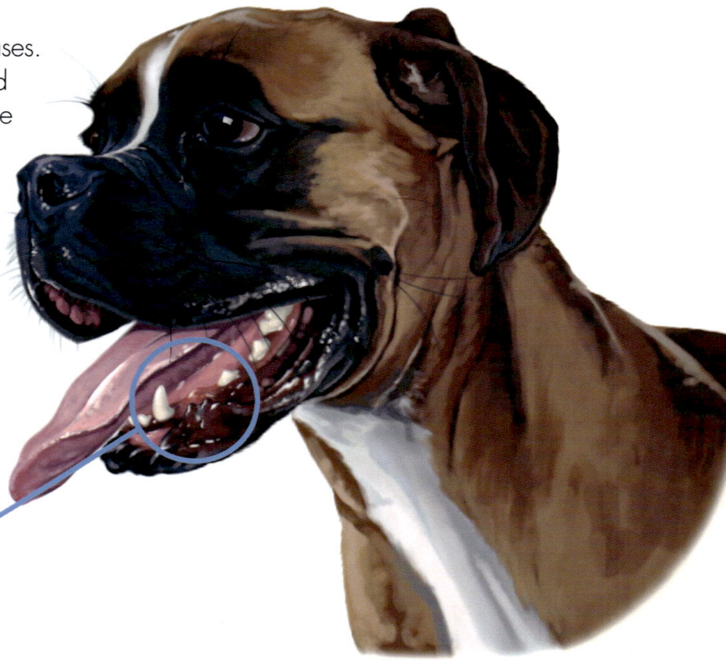

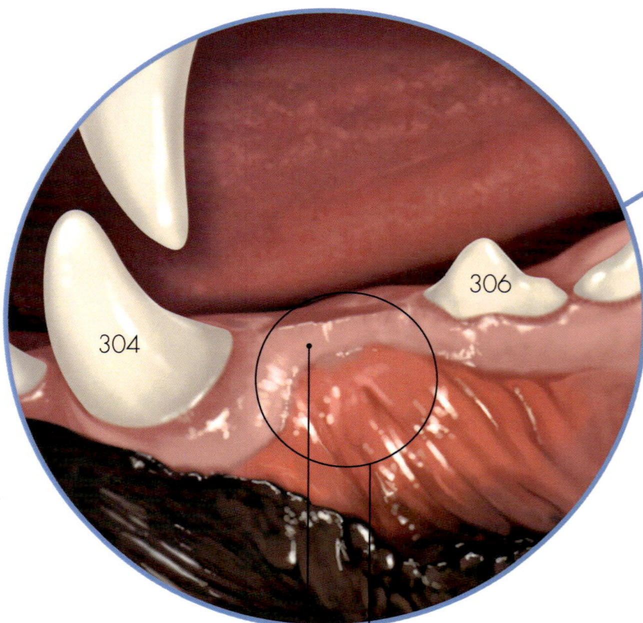

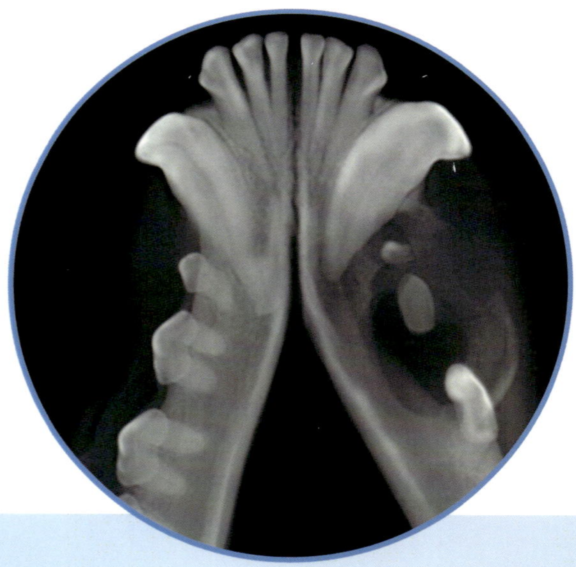

Brachycephalic dogs such as Boxers often develop dentigerous cysts associated with eruption failure of the mandibular first premolar.

Treatment

Dentigerous cysts are often diagnosed late, when their size is already externally detectable, at 2–3 years of age. Thus, it is advisable to make sure that all the teeth are present during the first visits to the veterinarian; if any are absent, an intraoral radiograph should be taken.

Preventive extraction of unerupted teeth is recommended to avoid the formation of these odontogenic cysts. However, in some cases, it is also possible to extrude the tooth using orthodontic techniques.

24 Alterations in enamel formation

Enamel formation can be affected in a generalized manner by various genetic, congenital, developmental, acquired, and nutritional diseases. Enamel defects limited to a single tooth or a specific area may be the result of trauma or infection in that area during enamel formation when the dog was a puppy.

This problem can affect a single tooth or several teeth. Within the same tooth, there may be areas with healthy enamel and other areas with defective or damaged, fragile, and brittle enamel.

Affected animals require periodic treatment, so daily tooth brushing by the owner is even more important in these cases to delay the need for ultrasonic scaling under general anesthesia.

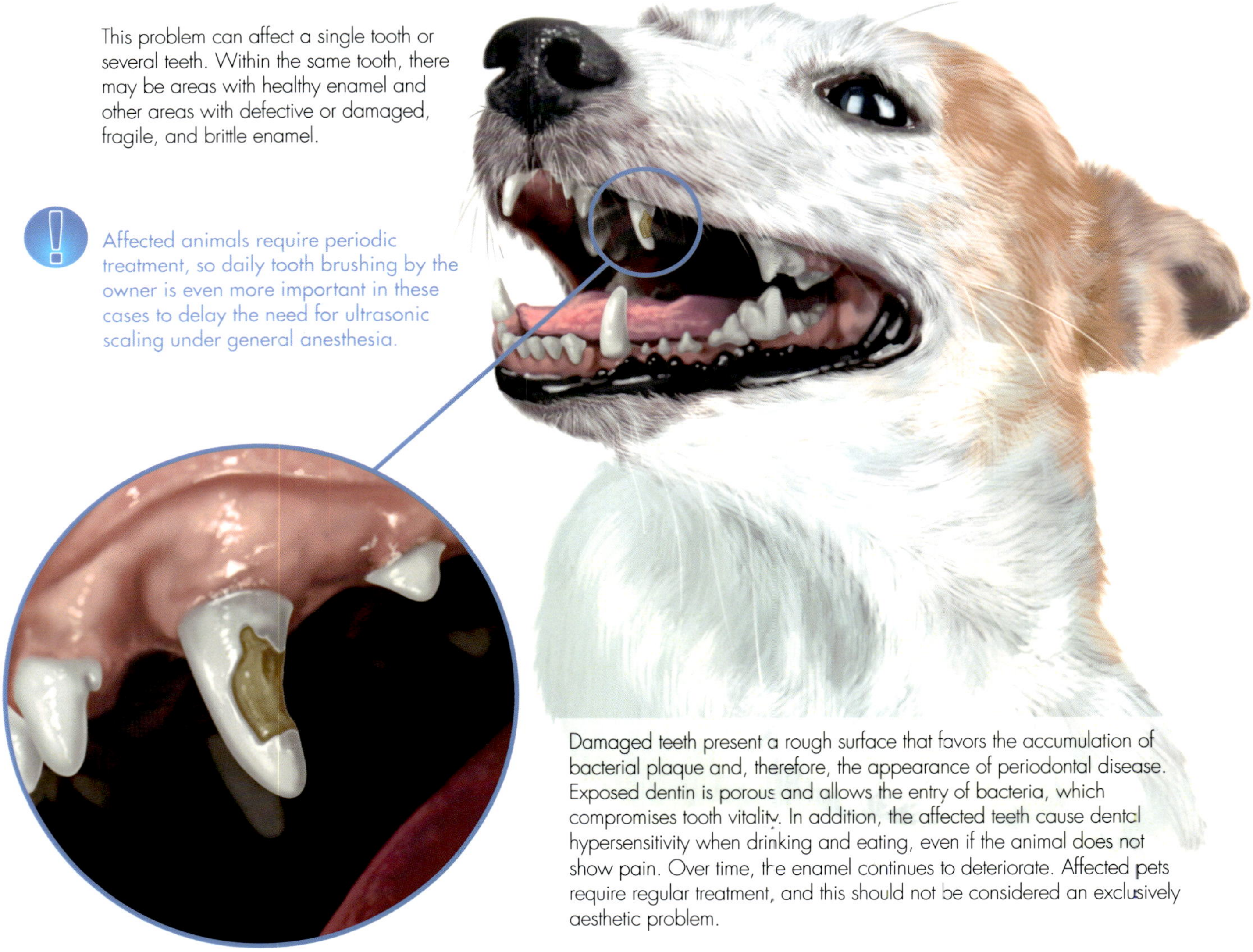

Damaged teeth present a rough surface that favors the accumulation of bacterial plaque and, therefore, the appearance of periodontal disease. Exposed dentin is porous and allows the entry of bacteria, which compromises tooth vitality. In addition, the affected teeth cause dental hypersensitivity when drinking and eating, even if the animal does not show pain. Over time, the enamel continues to deteriorate. Affected pets require regular treatment, and this should not be considered an exclusively aesthetic problem.

Treatment

- Intraoral radiography of all the teeth. Reevaluation at 6 months to assess tooth maturation.
- Extraction of nonvital teeth.
- The exposed dentin of vital teeth must be sealed to prevent bacterial penetration and subsequent pulpitis. Sealing also decreases tooth hypersensitivity.
- Important teeth, such as canines, can be restored with composite to achieve a smooth surface that does not retain bacterial plaque, or even with a prosthetic crown to avoid possible fractures.
- Professional cleaning should be carried out manually and with special care, otherwise the enamel may be further damaged.

25 Dental fractures

Tooth fractures may affect only the enamel or can reach the cementum and pulp. They should be assessed radiologically to establish the appropriate treatment.

Most dental fractures go unnoticed by owners until they cause a serious infection.

Classification of dental fractures

1. **Enamel fracture:** Small infraction or breakage that only affects the enamel.
2. **Uncomplicated crown fracture:** The enamel and dentin are affected, but the pulp is not exposed.
3. **Complicated crown fracture:** The enamel and dentin are affected, and the pulp is exposed.
4. **Uncomplicated crown and root fracture:** The enamel, dentin, and cementum are affected, but the pulp is not exposed.
5. **Complicated crown and root fracture:** The enamel, dentin, and cementum are affected, and the pulp is exposed.
6. **Root fracture:** The enamel, cementum, and pulp are affected.

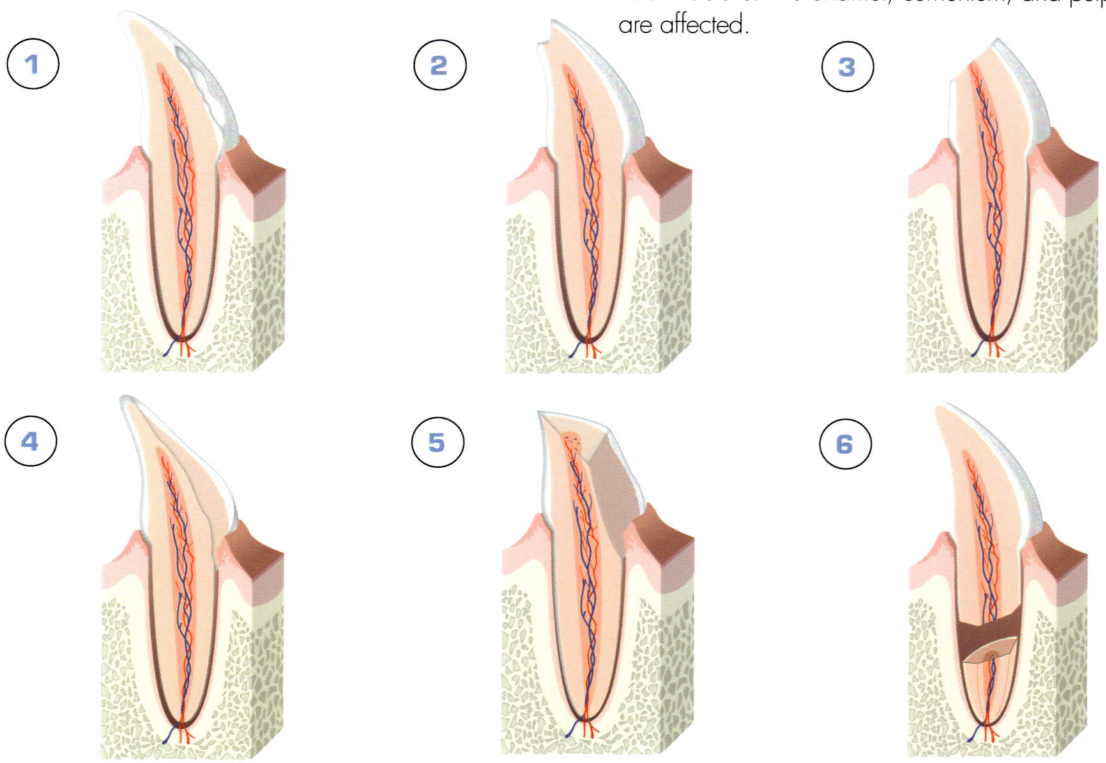

Treatment

- **Fractures that do not affect the pulp canal (uncomplicated)** can be restored with composite (filling) to avoid sensitivity and to maintain tooth vitality (exposed dentin is porous and in the long term can compromise tooth vitality). Some fractures leave sharp edges on the tooth that can cause mucosal damage (see Sheet 39).
- **Fractures involving the pulp canal (complicated)** always require treatment, either by extraction or, when possible, conservative treatment of the tooth through endodontics (see Sheets 39 and 42).
- These fractures can cause severe infection and pain in the animal, although their manifestations may go unnoticed.

26 Pathogenesis of periapical lesions

Complicated fractures affect the pulp canal (blood vessels and nerve). At the beginning, bleeding is observed and the tooth is very painful, although these signs can go unnoticed. Afterwards, the nerve dies and the root canal infection reaches the apex and destroys the periapical bone (which will be radiologically visible). This situation can progress to form a granuloma, cyst, or abscess (which is extremely painful). These lesions are often only detected when externally visible, indicating that the animal has had the infection for a long time.

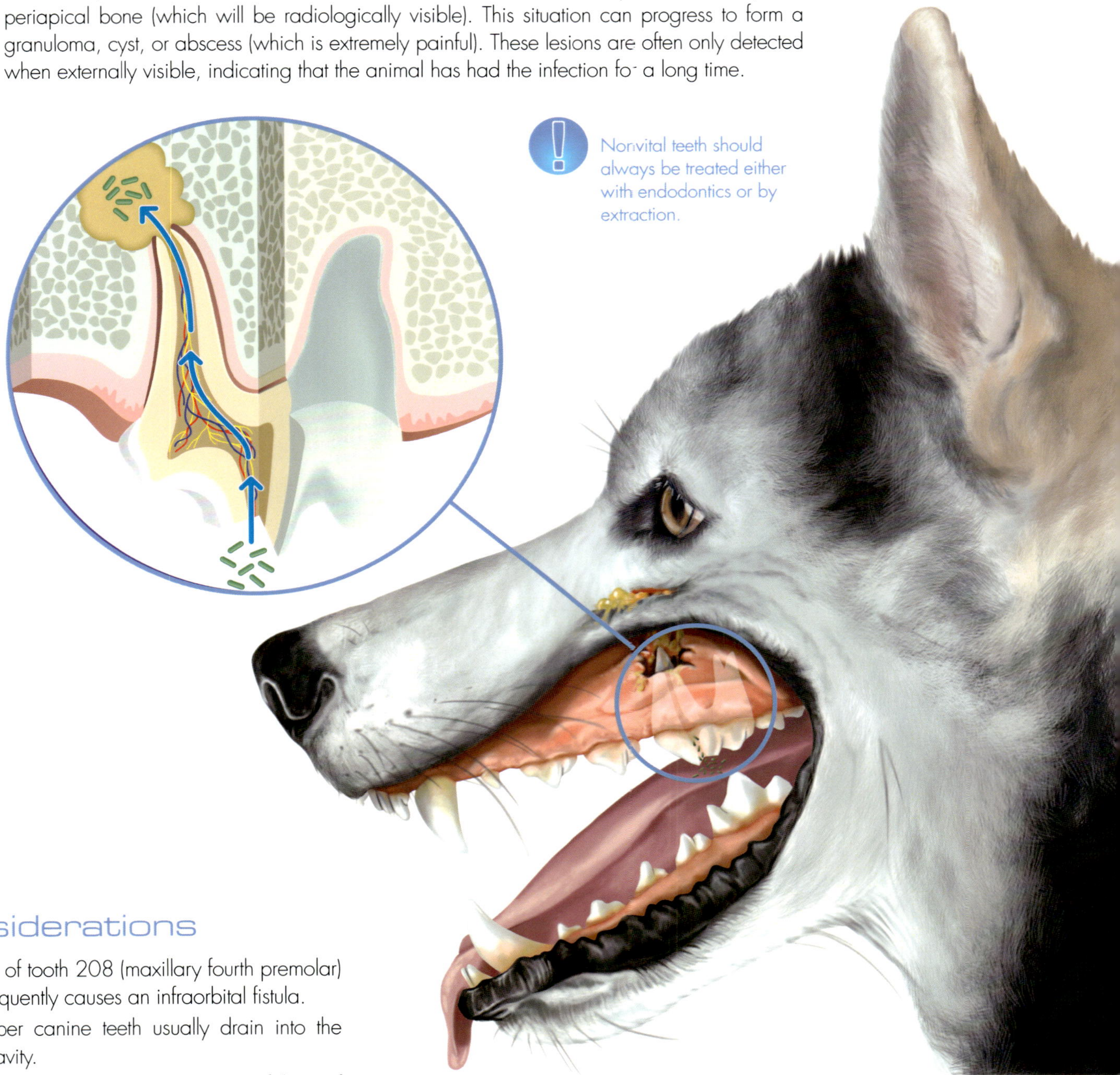

Nonvital teeth should always be treated either with endodontics or by extraction.

Considerations

- Fracture of tooth 208 (maxillary fourth premolar) most frequently causes an infraorbital fistula.
- The upper canine teeth usually drain into the nasal cavity.
- One of the most common causes of loss of tooth vitality is a crown fracture, although it can also occur in teeth with an intact crown due to occult periodontitis (see Sheets 14–16) or trauma without crown fracture (see Sheet 27).

The use of antibiotics as the sole treatment encourages lesions to persist because they mask, but do not resolve, the pathology.

27 Tooth color changes

The most frequent cause of localized tooth color changes is usually a blow or trauma. Other causes include genetic disorders, systemic diseases, and the ingestion of certain medications, such as tetracyclines, during tooth development; in these cases, discoloration will affect all the teeth.

When a tooth is subjected to a blow or trauma, even if no fracture is observed externally, the pulp blood vessels become inflamed and can rupture. Inflammation of the pulp (pulpitis) often results in pulp necrosis, with loss of tooth vitality and bacterial infection of the dental pulp.

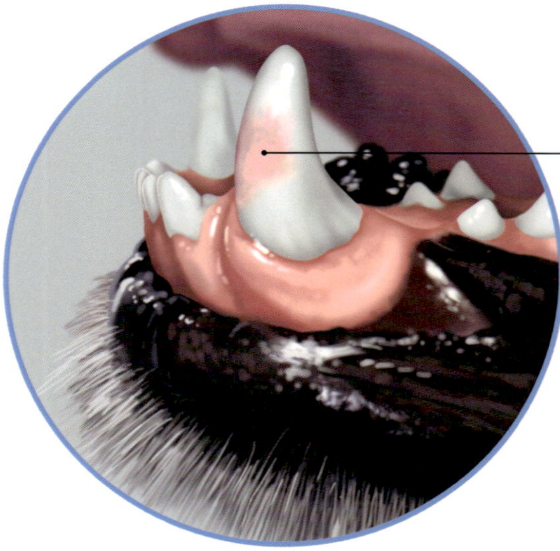

Initially, a **pinkish color** is observed
Reversible pulpitis
Treatment: Anti-inflammatories and analgesics to reduce the pressure inside the tooth and control pain

Any change in tooth color should be investigated by intraoral radiography to assess tooth vitality. The treatment of choice is endodontics or extraction.

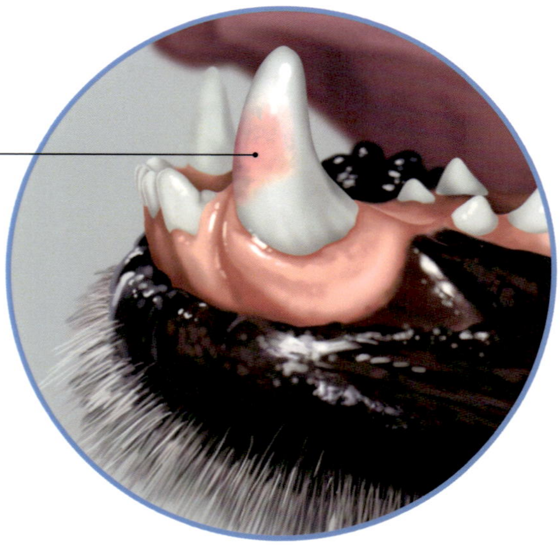

The hematoma evolves to a **purplish color** as blood cell decomposition begins
Irreversible pulpitis, in most cases
Treatment: Endodontics or extraction

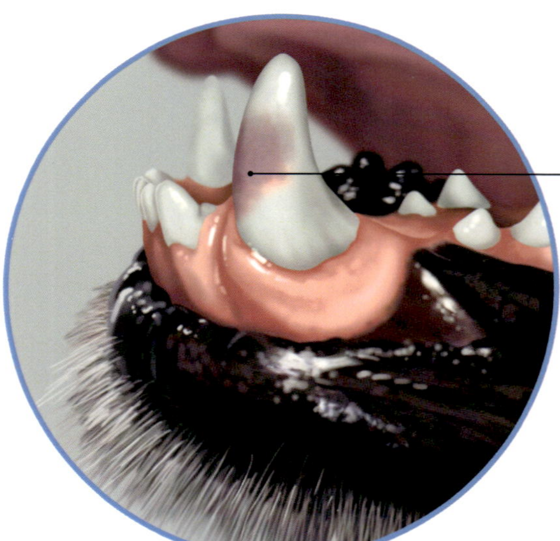

A **grayish color** indicates an older lesion, with pulp necrosis: partial or total death of the dental pulp
Treatment: Endodontics or extraction

Most animals do not show pain, so careful attention should be paid to any changes in tooth color.

28 Attrition and abrasion

Attrition is the wear that occurs when two teeth rub against each other, and it is more pronounced in the case of malocclusion or dental crowding. **Abrasion** is the wear of the tooth, both by normal use and by contact with hard objects such as tennis balls, stones, sticks, or cage bars.

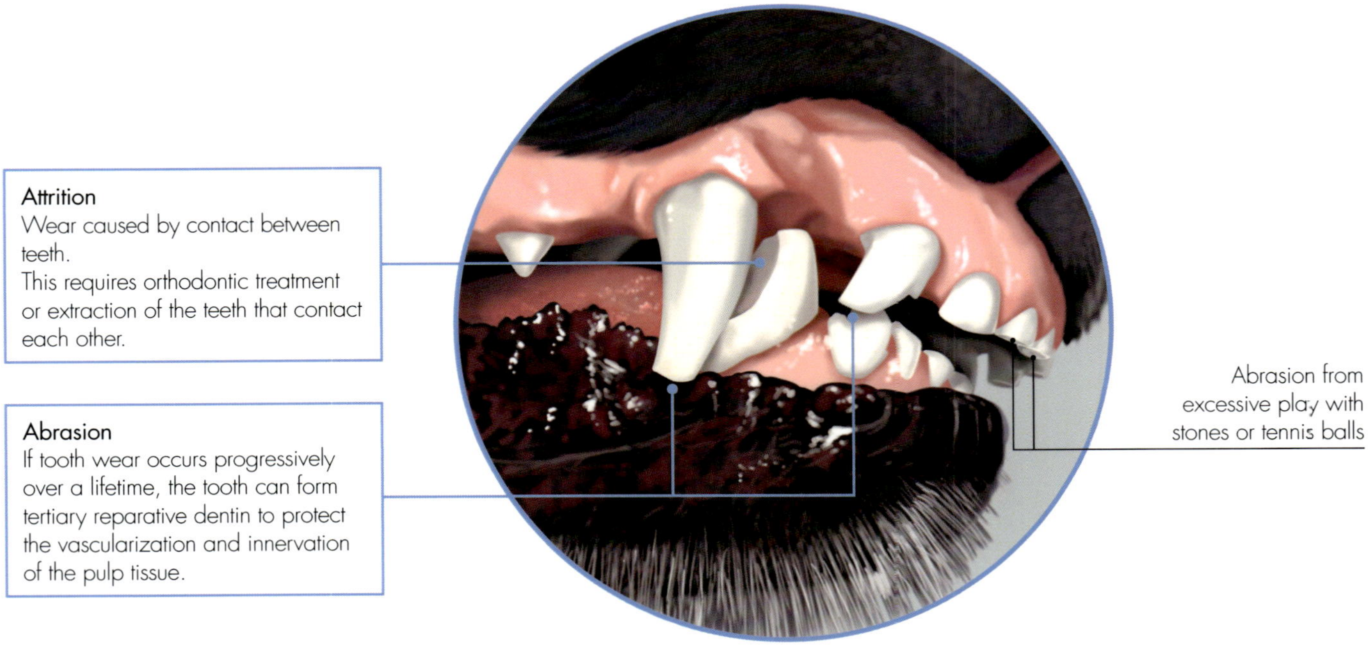

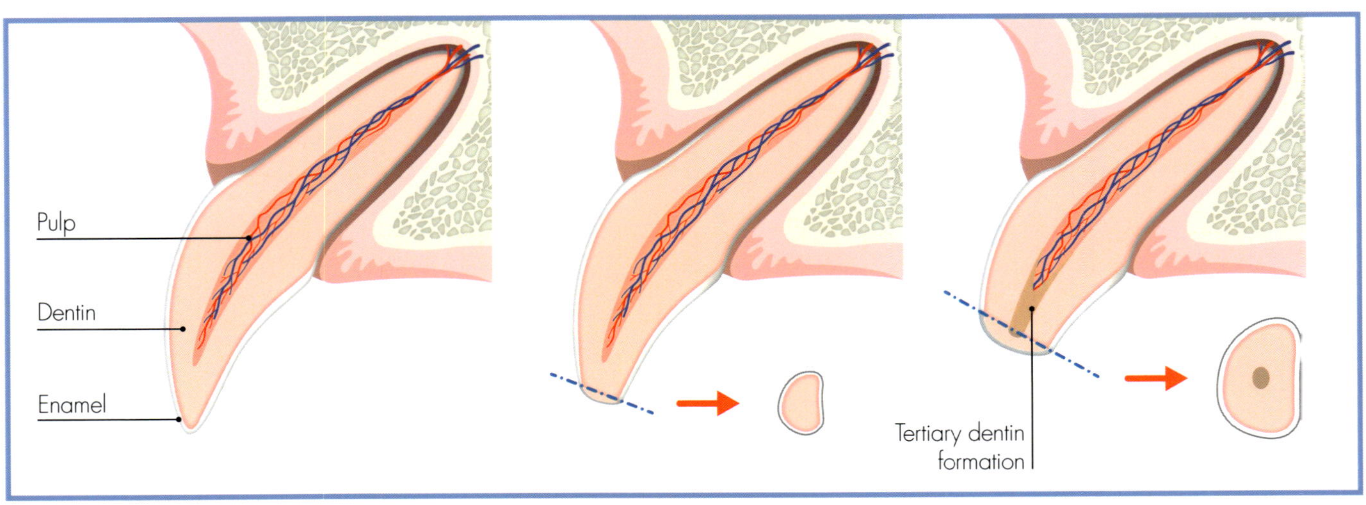

Treatment

- **Abrasion due to normal wear:** Abrasion with appropriate tertiary dentin formation does not require treatment if intraoral radiography shows that the tooth is healthy.
- **Abrasion caused by excessive use or play with hard objects:** When tooth wear occurs faster than the tooth's ability to produce tertiary reparative dentin, the pulp may become inflamed or even exposed, causing the loss of tooth vitality. In these cases, extraction or root canal therapy (endodontics) is required (see Sheets 39 and 42, respectively).

29 Best practices to avoid abrasion

There are numerous options for toys designed to stimulate play in cats and dogs without damaging their teeth. This helps to prevent them from playing with sticks and stones they may find in parks or from chewing dangerous objects, such as wires in the case of cats.

The best toys for chewing and playing should be made of materials that are not too hard to avoid fractures and dental abrasion but that are strong so that they do not easily break into pieces that could be accidentally swallowed.

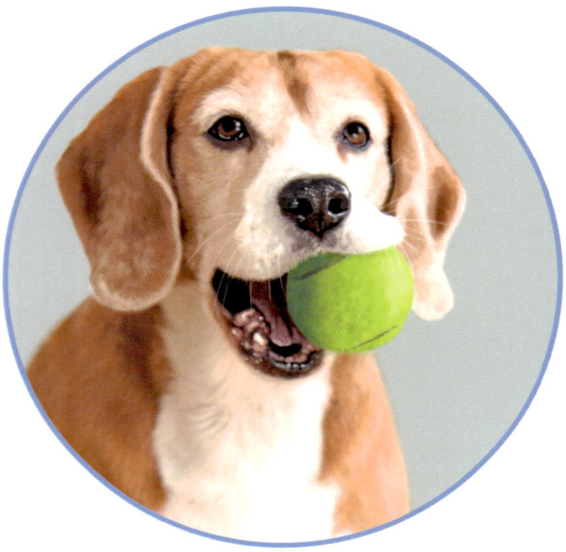

Tennis balls are made of very abrasive materials. Dogs that usually play with these balls often suffer excessive wear of the teeth.

If the wear is faster than the ability of the odontoblasts in the dental pulp to produce reparative dentin, the pulp may become inflamed or even exposed, causing the loss of tooth vitality.

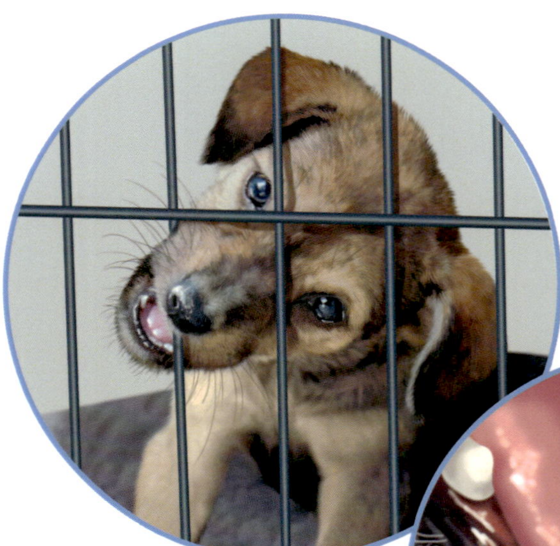

Some dogs may bite the bars of their enclosures or crates when they are confined. Abrasion from biting these bars produces characteristic wear on the distal aspect of the canines.

Excessive play with hard objects and traumatic occlusion also lead to resorption of the dental roots (see Sheet 32).

Enamel loss exposes the dentin, whose more porous structure means bacteria can get into it more easily, with subsequent pulp necrosis. In addition, excessive loss of tooth structure predisposes animals to crown fractures.

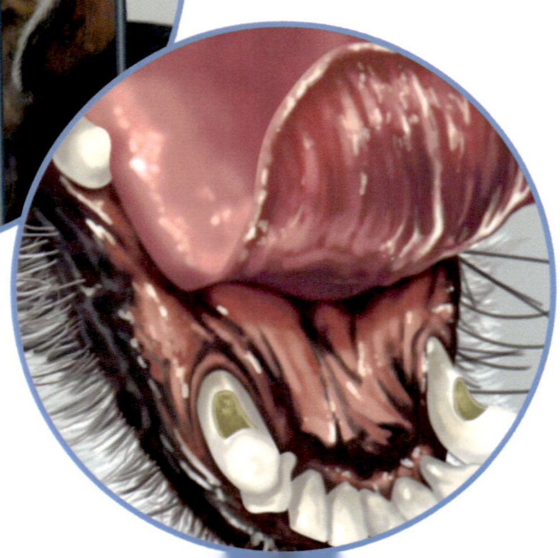

30 Caries

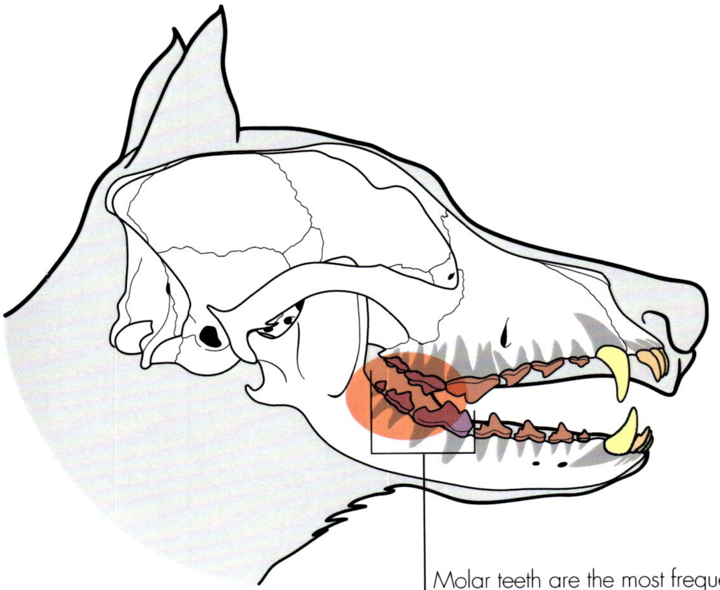

Molar teeth are the most frequent location of caries in cats and dogs, although any other tooth can be affected

Caries (cavities) are rare in dogs. They are caused by bacteria that feed on carbohydrates and sugars. This explains why these lesions are so frequent in people and so infrequent in carnivores.

In addition, the crowns of the teeth of cats and dogs are adapted to cut food, and their shape makes it difficult for food debris to adhere to them. The exception is molar teeth, as their occlusal aspect is flat (cariogenic surface), where the accumulation of bacterial plaque and food debris is more frequent, favoring the development of caries.

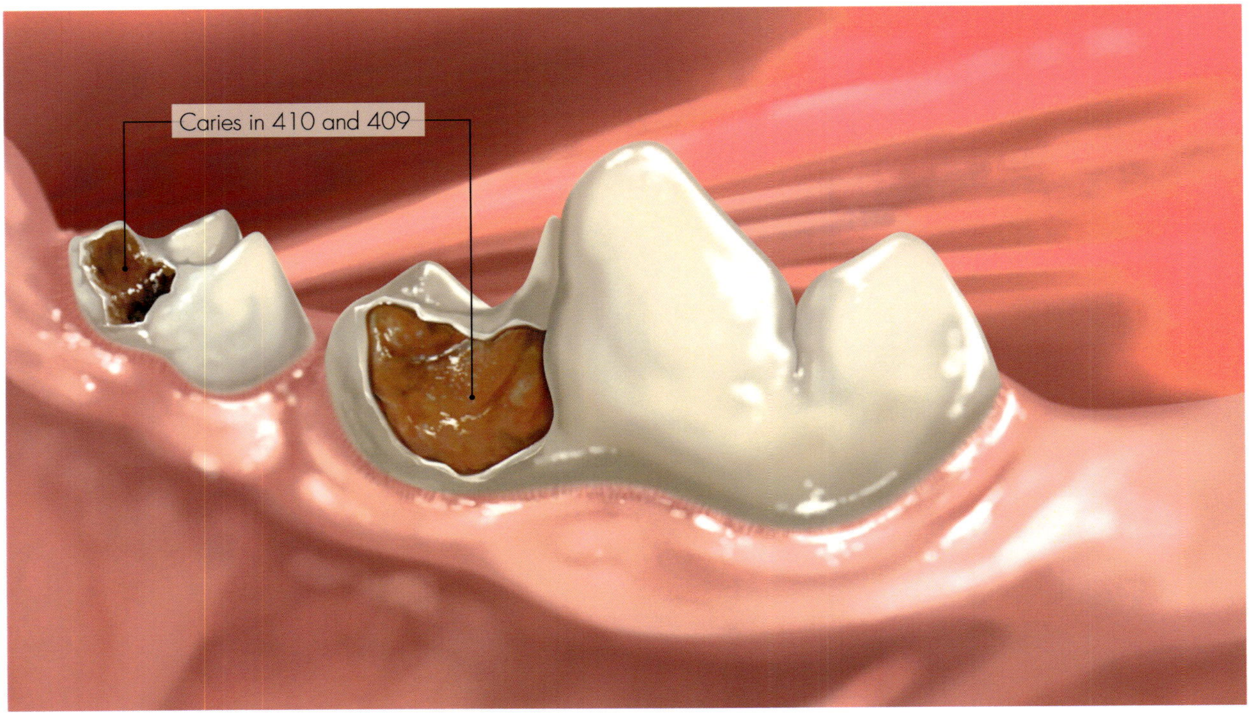

Caries often occur in animals fed with table scraps, as this food is usually rich in sugars and carbohydrates (cariogenic diet).

Treatment

Removal of the damaged tooth surface and restoration. Deeper caries affecting the pulp require endodontics or extraction (see Sheets 42 and 39, respectively).

31 Resorptive lesions in cats

These lesions are the most frequent dental pathology found in domestic cats. Up to 70% of cats suffer from this disease during their lifetime and the frequency of presentation increases with age, although these lesions are infrequent in cats under 2 years of age. The cause is still unknown and probably multifactorial, but cats fed a high-quality diet and whose owners brush their teeth have fewer lesions.

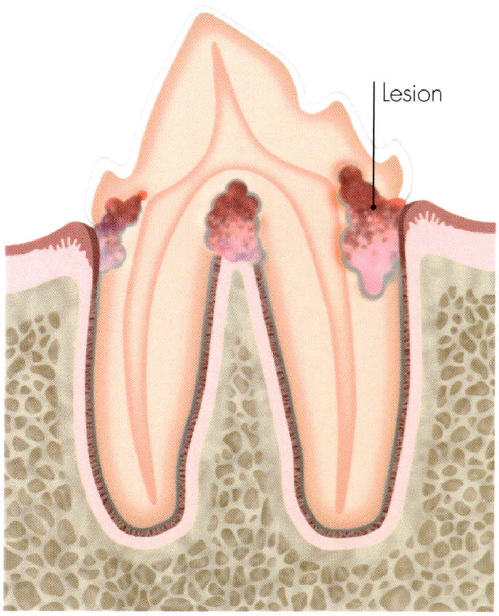

Lesions can appear in any part of the tooth but are more frequent in the cervical area (between the root and the crown) and in the furcation (between the roots).

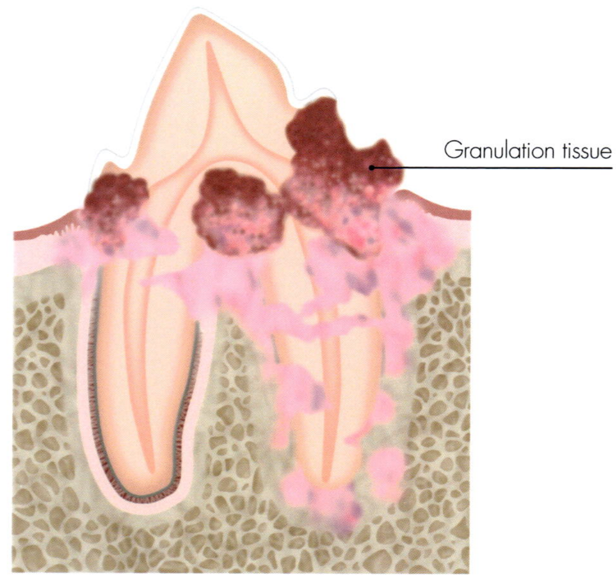

Advanced lesions in the cervical area are covered by granulation tissue as a protective mechanism. They can be clinically observed by the veterinarian during examination.

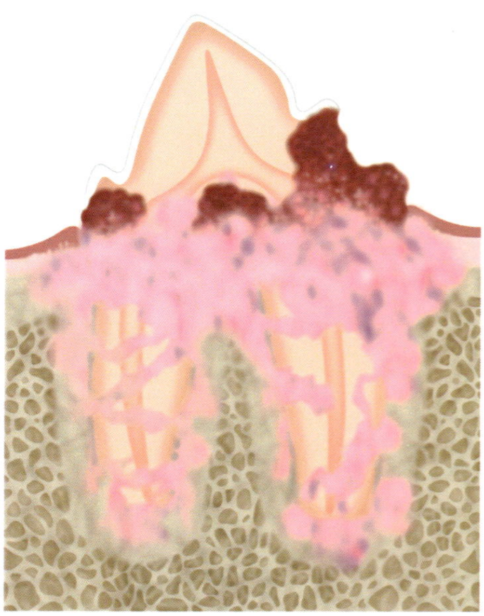

As the disease progresses, the lesions below the gingival margin and in the roots (undetectable) increase.

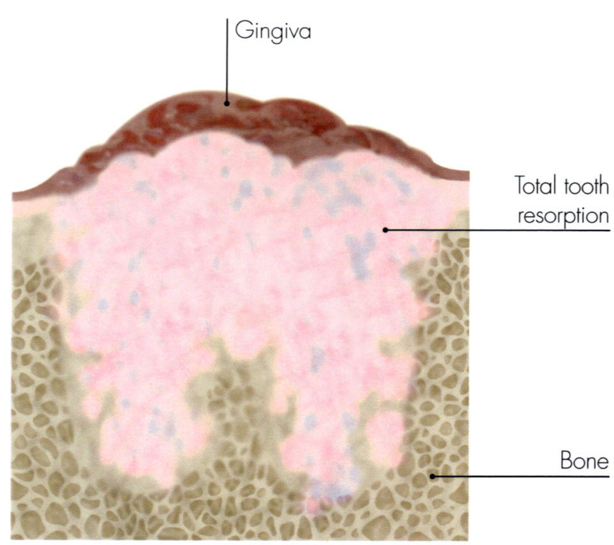

The disease progresses until the tooth is completely resorbed. Crown fractures and root remnants are common.

Clinical signs

The onset of these lesions is usually asymptomatic, but when resorption progresses to the nerve endings of the dental pulp, the disorder is very painful. The owner may notice that the cat drops food from their mouth, refuses cold water, prefers a soft food diet, has chattering teeth, hypersalivates, or shows signs of apathy.

Cats that spontaneously lose any teeth should be examined under general anesthesia, because it is very likely that they will have more lesions.

Any tooth can be affected, but lesions in mandibular teeth, especially in the third premolar, are frequent. Bilateral symmetrical lesions are often observed. Signs of periodontitis, such as gingival recession and inflammation and loss of tooth support, as well as tooth extrusion and buccal bone expansion are also often simultaneously found.

Buccal bone expansion is a thickening of the alveolar bone associated with periodontitis. It is exclusively found in cats, and the cause is unknown.

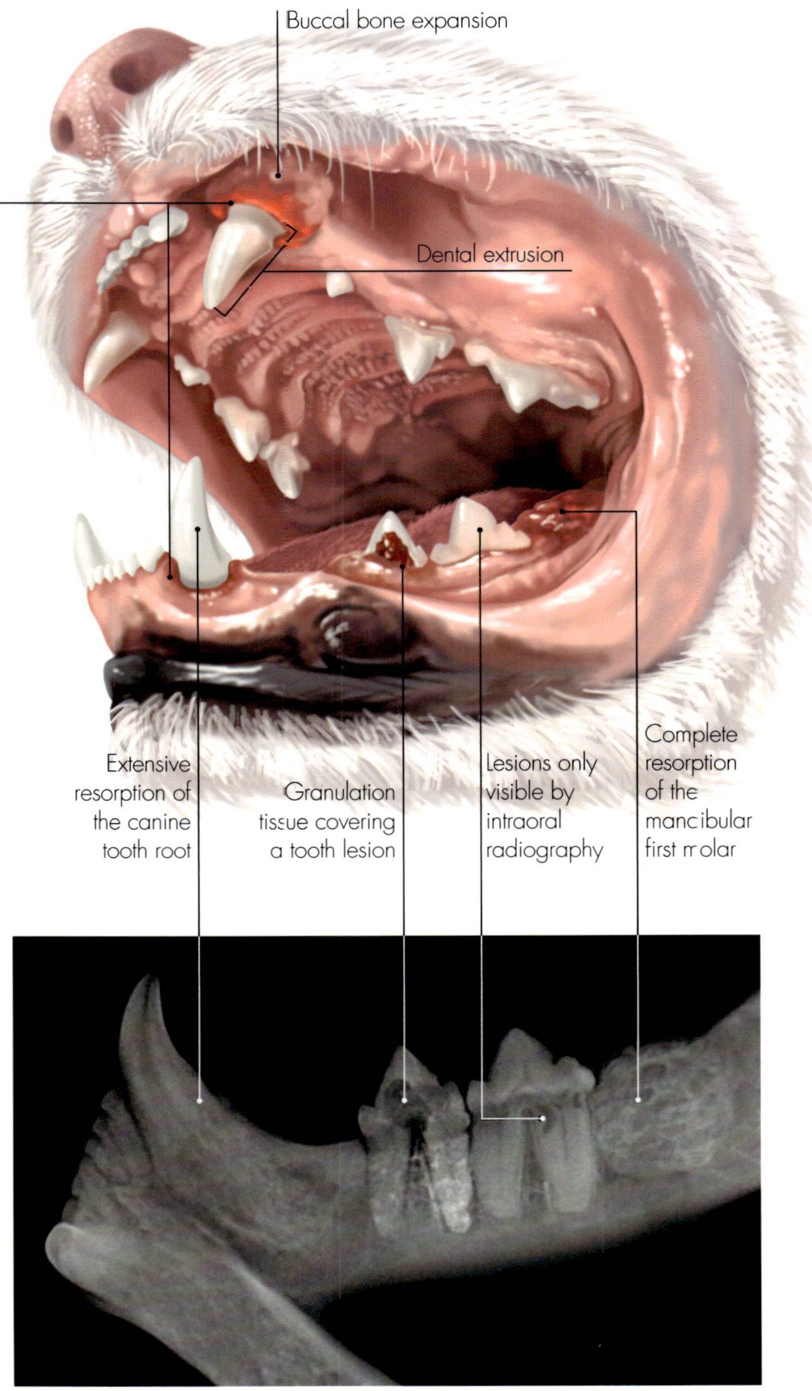

Given the frequency of resorptive lesions in cats, a complete intraoral radiological study must be performed before any oral treatment is applied.

Crown lesions are usually covered by a characteristic layer of granulation tissue which can be easily observed by routine examination of the mouth. There is a high likelihood that other occult lesions will also be present.

Resorptive lesions are often found in conjunction with periodontitis and feline stomatitis.

Most lesions are located below the gingival margin and are not clinically detectable, so performing a complete intraoral radiological study is essential (see Sheet 13).

Treatment

The appropriate treatment for affected teeth is complete extraction. Healthy teeth may develop the disease later, and so it is advisable to perform a checkup every 6 months to detect new lesions early on.

32 Resorptive lesions in dogs

Some dental resorption processes are physiological, such as during deciduous tooth exfoliation. However, in adulthood, tooth resorption is considered pathological because it affects the permanent teeth. Of note, up to 50% of dogs present this type of lesion in one or more teeth.

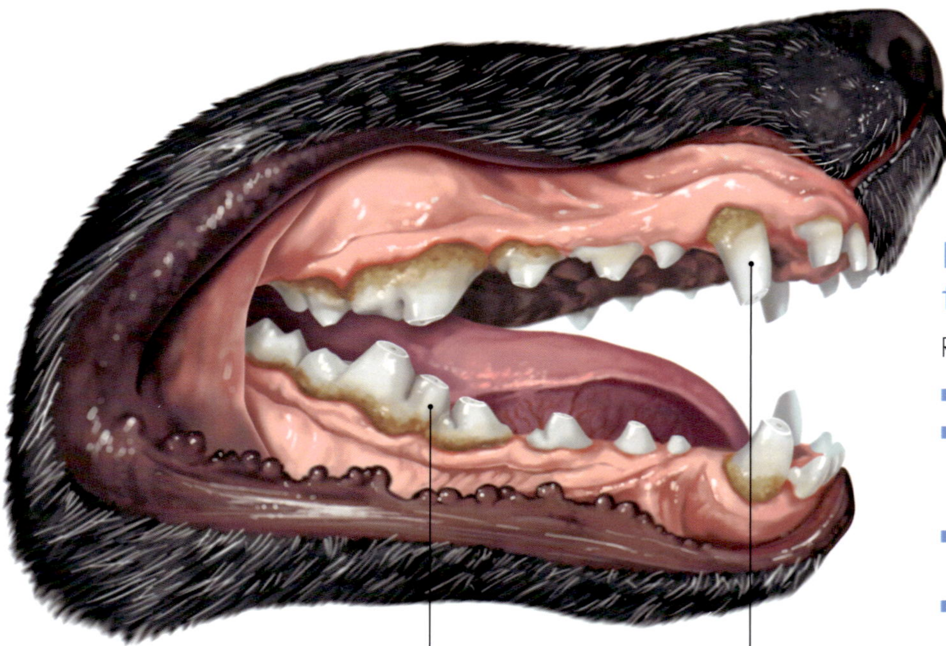

Resorptive lesions may be an indicator of the presence of oral cavity neoplasms.

Predisposing factors

Resorptive lesions are more common in:

- Large-sized breeds.
- Older dogs, although they are usually asymptomatic and do not require treatment if the crown is intact.
- Dogs with the habit of biting hard objects (see Sheet 28).
- Teeth with periodontitis or endodontic pathology.
- Dogs with systemic diseases.
- Animals with dental trauma (tooth luxation and avulsion).
- Dogs with oral neoplasms.

If the crown or pulp is affected, or if resorption is associated with periodontitis, the treatment should be tooth extraction.

These lesions are classified according to their extent and radiographic appearance. Intraoral radiography is required to diagnose and characterize the different types of lesions and to provide appropriate treatment. External replacement resorption and external inflammatory resorption are the most common resorptive lesions in dogs. Furthermore, some lesions may be progressive in nature, cause pain, and predispose dogs to spontaneous crown fractures; thus treatment is warranted.

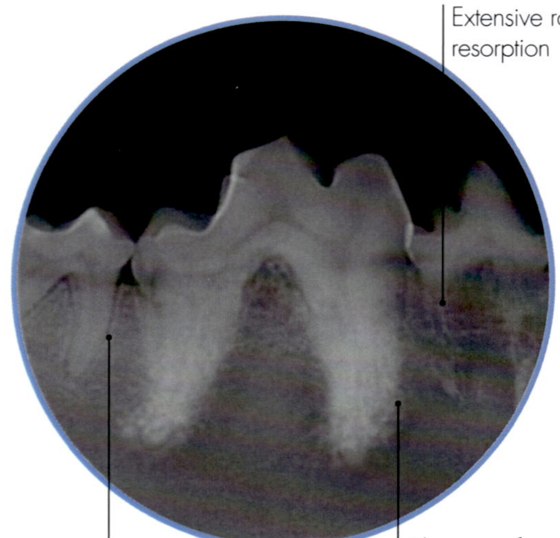

33 Ulcerative stomatitis in dogs

Also called ulcerative paradental stomatitis or contact mucosal ulceration, this is an oral inflammatory disease in dogs characterized by the appearance of ulcers on the oral mucosa in areas that contact the surface of the teeth. The etiology is not completely known, but, like in feline gingivostomatitis, an abnormal immune system response to bacterial plaque is involved. Cocker Spaniels and, in general, medium-sized breeds are more prone to this disorder.

Careful examination

Severe halitosis is often the initial presenting complaint. During examination, the lip should be carefully lifted because these ulcers are very painful (in the most severe cases, tissue necrosis occurs). Lesions are observed on the mucosa in contact with teeth with periodontitis, but they may also appear associated with healthy teeth due to daily accumulation of bacterial plaque.

Risk zones

The areas most frequently affected are the mucosa in contact with the canine teeth and with the maxillary carnassial tooth, areas where the most bacterial plaque accumulates. However, ulcerative stomatitis can also affect the mucosa in contact with any other tooth, the lateral margins of the tongue, and the labial commissure.

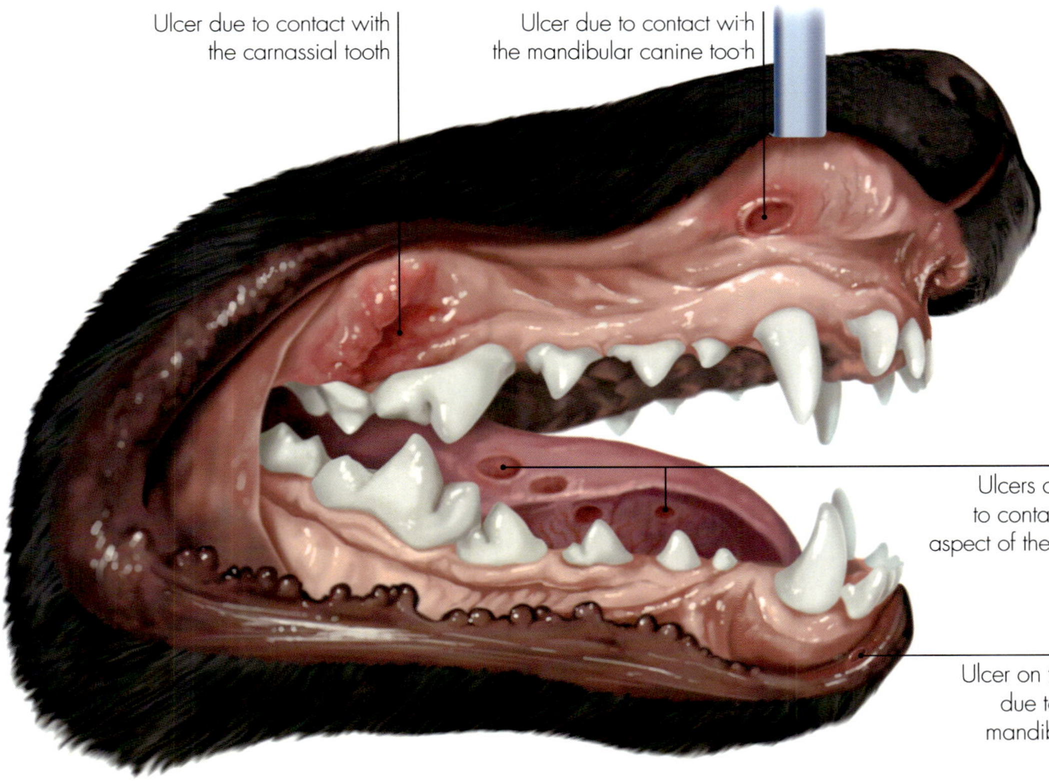

Treatment

Mild cases can initially be managed with ultrasonic scaling, polishing, and treatment of any teeth with periodontitis. However, the active participation and commitment of the owner in daily brushing of their pet's teeth is essential in the long term because the accumulation of bacterial plaque will trigger the appearance of ulcers again in the future.

Antibiotic therapy is not an alternative to daily tooth brushing and is not effective in the long-term control of this disease. When daily oral hygiene is not possible or is insufficient, extraction of the teeth involved is the treatment of choice.

34 Feline chronic gingivostomatitis

Feline chronic gingivostomatitis is a severe inflammatory disease affecting the gums (gingivitis) and oral mucosa (mucositis). This condition is very painful and limits the cat's quality of life.

The primary cause is unknown, but numerous factors may be involved. An abnormal and exaggerated immune response to infectious antigens (such as plaque bacteria and viruses) occurs, and external factors such as stress may play a role. Affected cats suffer from severe pain and have difficulty eating.

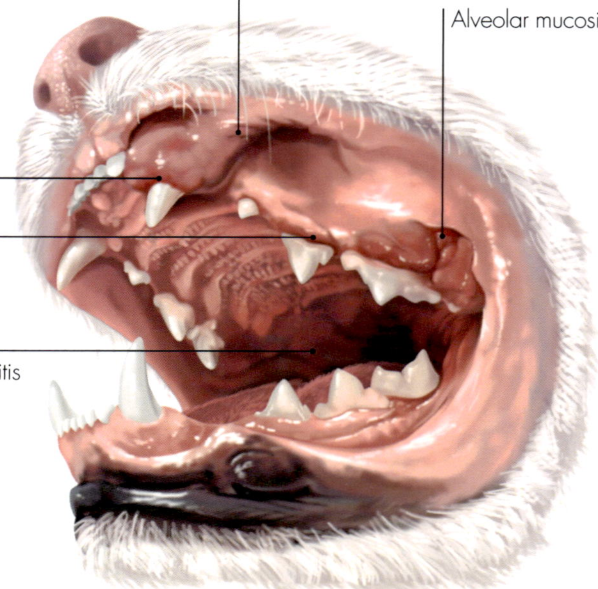

Caudal mucositis

Diagnosis is based on the clinical presentation and location of the lesions: gingivitis and alveolar, buccal, and caudal mucositis.

Caudal mucositis is ulceration of the mucosa lateral to the palatoglossal arches and is a characteristic lesion of this disease, although it may not initially be present.

Chronic cases are more severe: the lesions are worse, and proliferative tissue and even ulcers on the tongue can be observed.

It is advisable to perform a serological analysis for FIV (immunodeficiency), FeLV (leukemia), FHV (herpesvirus), and FCV (calicivirus) as well as a complete blood analysis to assess the patient's general health status.

Diagnostic confirmation by biopsy is not usually necessary, although it is essential in proliferative or asymmetrical lesions.

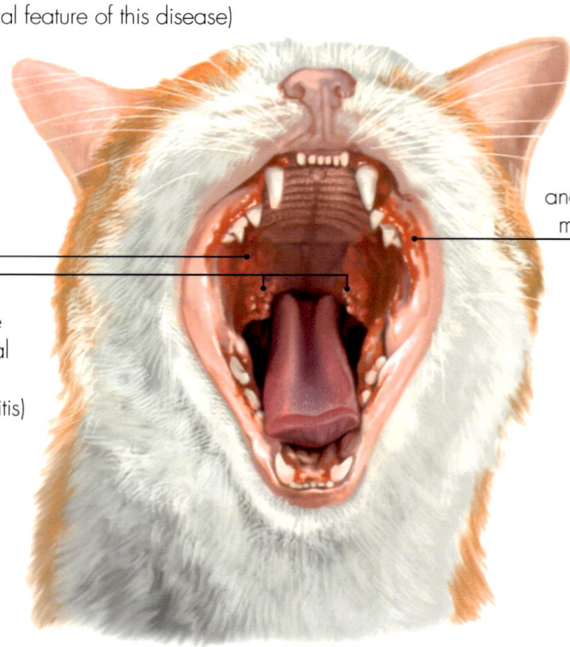

FCV is more frequently detected in cats affected by feline chronic gingivostomatitis but is not considered diagnostic for the disease.

Associated pathologies

Most cats affected with gingivostomatitis also have other dental pathologies. Therefore, before instituting any medical treatment, it is essential to perform a complete oral examination of the cat under general anesthesia, including periodontal probing and intraoral radiological assessment of all the teeth.

Dental pathologies that may be associated with this disease and that contribute to the persistence of oral inflammation are periodontal disease, tooth resorption, the presence of root remnants, and endodontic pathologies.

Surgical treatment

Selective extraction of premolars and molars

If the owner brushes the remaining pet's teeth (incisors and canines in this case) on a daily basis, the result may be complete resolution of the disease. However, if the owner stops brushing, the lesions will quickly reappear, and extraction of all the teeth should be considered.

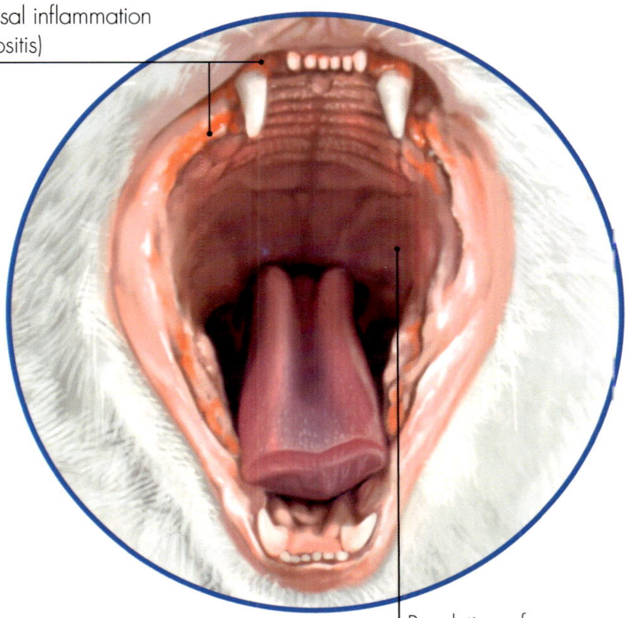

Medical treatment should be aimed at reducing oral inflammation and controlling pain (anti-inflammatory and analgesic drugs). The presence of any concomitant dental pathologies should be investigated and treated accordingly to prevent chronic oral inflammation.

Full mouth extraction

Without teeth, there is no plaque accumulation, so the altered immune response to plaque bacteria and, therefore, oral inflammation is reduced.

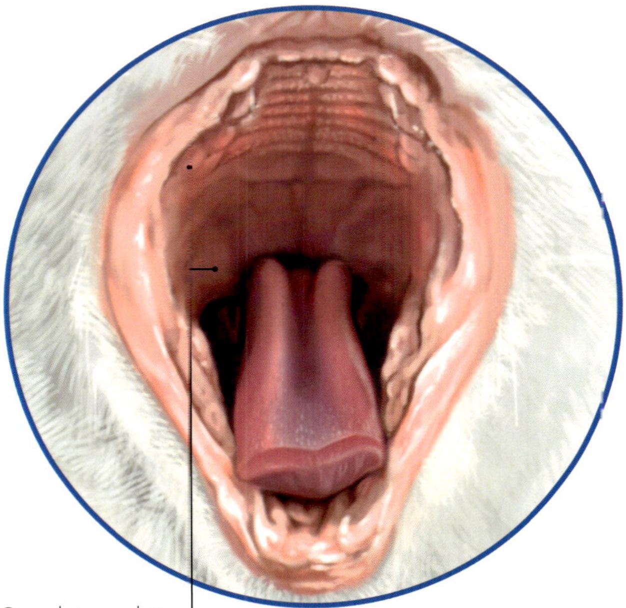

Negative prognostic factors

- Previous history of corticosteroid overuse.
- Delay in the necessary tooth extractions: the longer the decision is delayed, the more difficult it will be to achieve a positive response.
- Cats with proliferative lesions have a poorer prognosis because these are usually the consequence of long periods of medical treatment without a diagnosis of the underlying dental pathology.

Treatment

Up to 80% of cats improve fully or partially after dental extractions. Owners usually delay the decision to subject their cat to multiple extractions, but so far this still remains the only recommended treatment. The role of veterinarians is essential in transmitting information about the benefits of timely tooth extractions to owners.

Some cats require medical treatment after the extractions, and the most severe cases will need it for the rest of their lives.

35 Oronasal communication and palatal defects

Fissures and defects in the palate create communications between the mouth and nose. Any communication of the oral and nasal cavities allows bacteria from the mouth, and even food, to pass into the upper airways, resulting in clinical signs such as sneezing, coughing, purulent nasal discharge, and, in severe cases, pneumonia.

Palatal fissures and defects may be congenital (present at birth or caused by alterations during fetal development), acquired (consequence of trauma, such as fights, road traffic accidents, or falling from a height), secondary to untreated chronic periodontal disease (see Sheets 14–16), or due to contact with the mandibular canines in cases of traumatic malocclusion (see Sheet 9).

Oronasal communication and fistula

When an oronasal communication persists over time, lining tissue proliferates around the defect, resulting in a fistula. This can occur, for example, because of extraction of the maxillary canine in cases of advanced periodontitis (see Sheet 17). This additional tissue must be surgically removed.

Miniature and toy breeds are more predisposed to develop periodontitis. To avoid this complication, the affected teeth should be surgically extracted before bone destruction becomes even greater.

To facilitate cleaning of the alveolar bone and removal of the epithelial lining of the fistula, the canine tooth should be surgically extracted via an open flap technique.

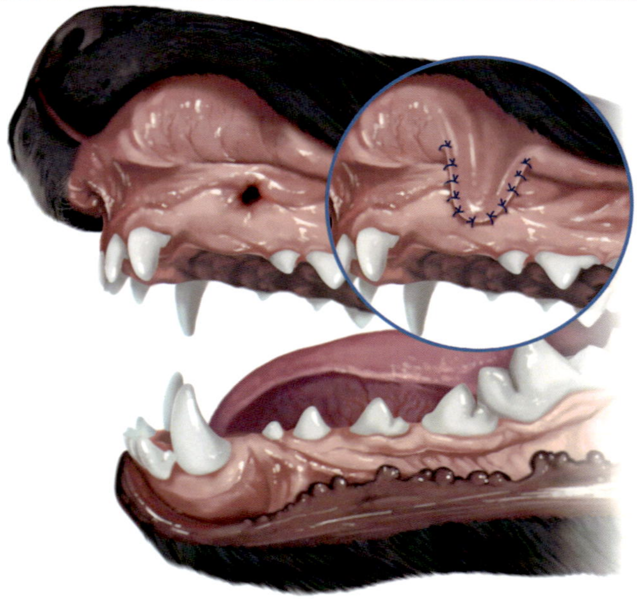

Cleft palate

Falls from a great height usually cause midline separation of the palate.

The surgical technique required to remediate this problem depends on the size and location of the defect.

Success is greater if the surgery is performed as soon as possible. Although some mild cases may resolve on their own, they should still be surgically corrected to avoid the formation of an oronasal fistula, which would be more complicated to treat.

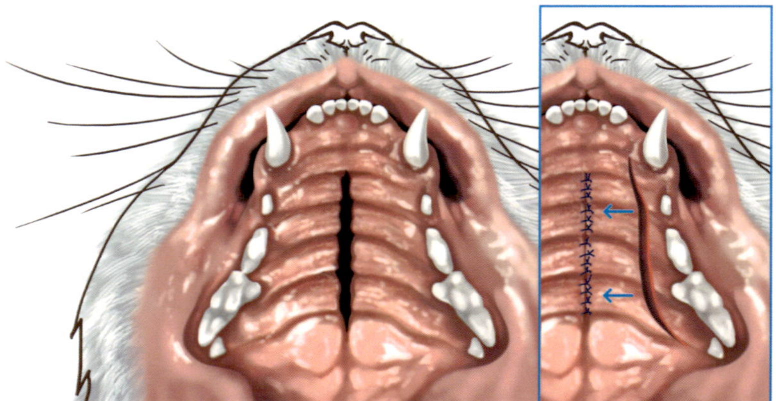

Diagnostic imaging

Intraoral radiology is useful to determine the extent of the bony defect, which is often larger than the externally visible defect. In this respect, computed tomography (CT) is a useful diagnostic tool both in cases of trauma, where other less apparent lesions are often found, and in cases of large defects and developmental abnormalities.

Tissues resulting from previous surgical attempts are weaker and may lack sufficient vascularization. Thus, surgery should be properly planned prior to any attempt at repair because poor execution will compromise the outcome of any subsequent interventions.

Large defects of the palate

Surgery

Large defects, whether congenital or acquired, require careful surgical planning because the availability of useful tissue is limited.

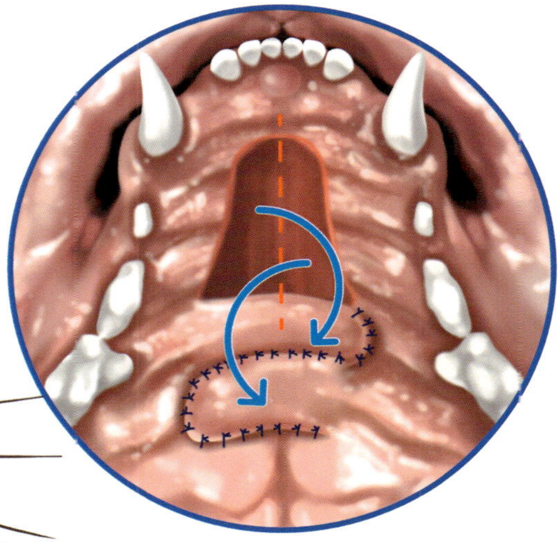

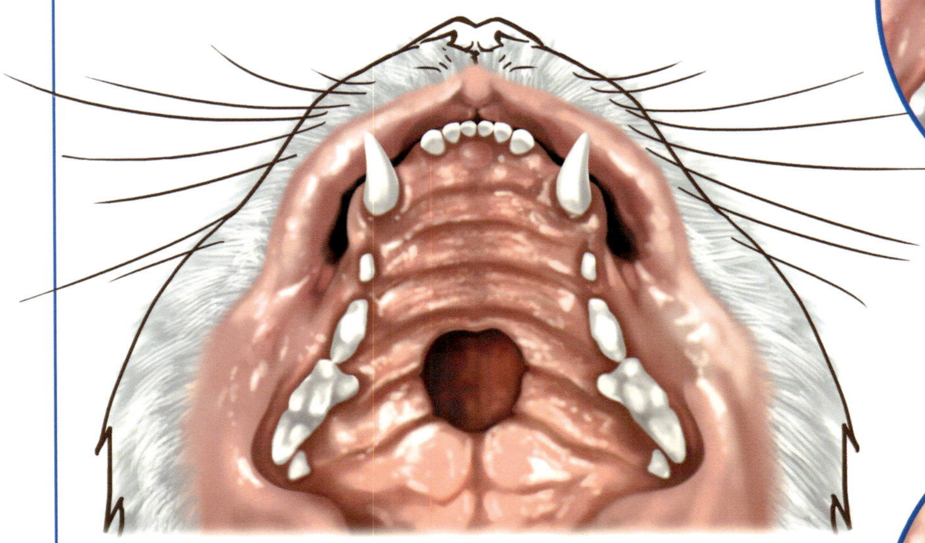

Temporary obturators

Temporary palatal obturators are used in the case of large defects and in puppies with congenital defects until they mature enough to undergo restorative surgery.

The successful repair of large defects depends on choosing the appropriate technique, the availability of tissue to make the repair, and the experience of the veterinary specialist.

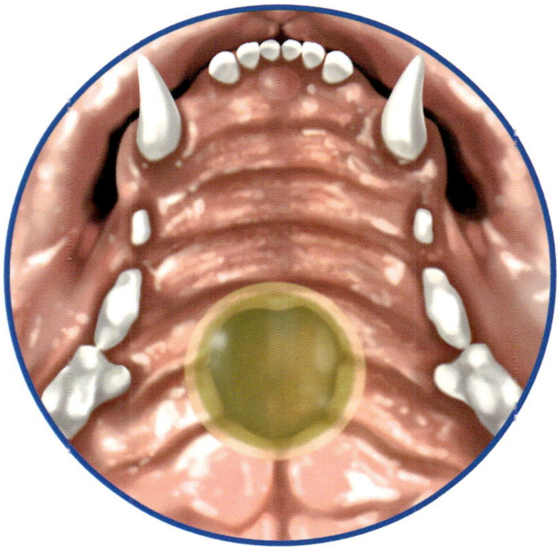

36 Oral neoplasms

Oral and maxillofacial neoplasms or tumors are common in cats and dogs. Those of the oral cavity are classified into odontogenic and nonodontogenic according to their origin and into benign and malignant according to their behavior.

Owners who brush their pet's teeth tend to detect any abnormalities present in the mouth earlier.

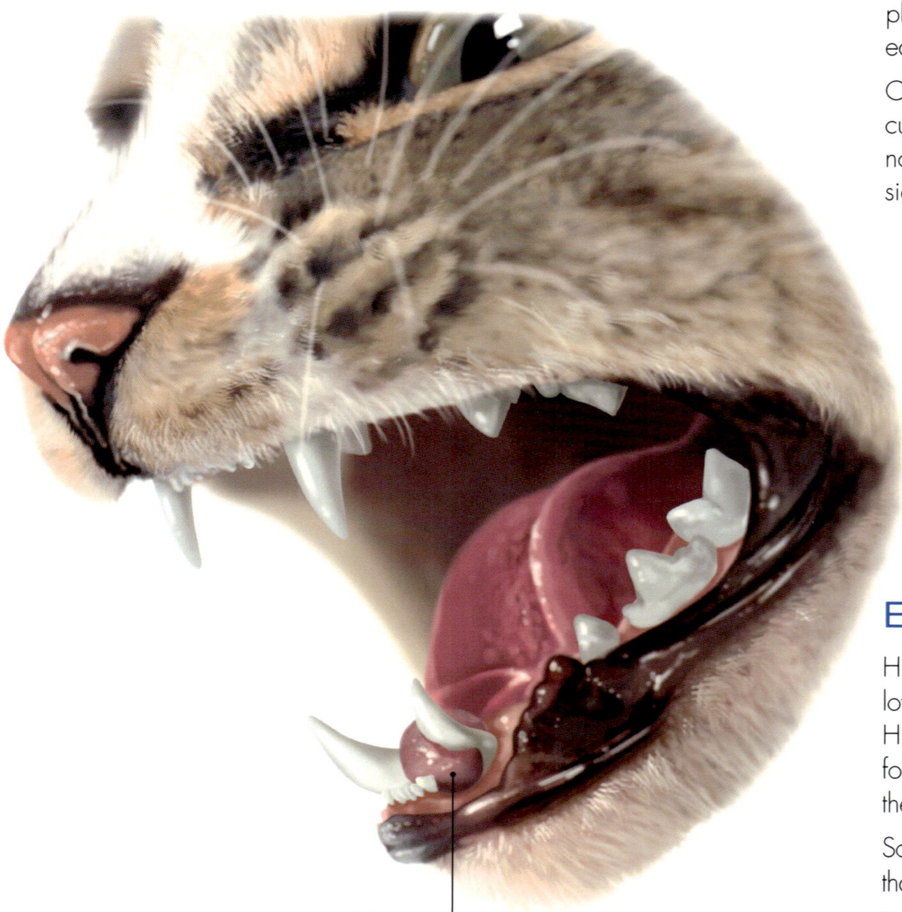

Early detection

Regular examination of the oral cavity during routine veterinary visits and palpation of regional lymph nodes are essential for the early detection of oral neoplasia.

The treatment success rate is higher for small neoplasms because it is easier to achieve tumor cell–free margins in these cases. Malignant neoplasms are more frequent in cats than in dogs, so early detection is even more important in felines.

Caudally located neoplasms are more difficult for owners to detect and so are often only noticed when they have already reached a considerable size.

Biopsy and cytology

Histopathological diagnosis by biopsy followed by cytological analysis is essential. Histopathological analysis should always be performed, regardless of the visual appearance of the lesions.

Some neoplasms present an atypical appearance that can easily be confused with periodontitis; for example, ulcerative lesions that do not heal or spontaneous tooth loss. A biopsy and cytological analysis should be performed for any mouth tissue alteration, even for apparently benign overgrowths such as gingival hyperplasia (see Sheet 41).

Planning

Intraoral radiography is essential to evaluate whether the bone is affected. Contrast computed tomography (CT) can be used to accurately determine the extent of the neoplasm and detect lymph node involvement and the presence of metastases, making its use indispensable to establish the appropriate treatment plan.

Benign oral neoplasms can reach a large size but do not form distant metastases. However, some are capable of infiltrating the underlying bone (bone invasion).

Oncological surgery

The objective of this treatment is to achieve rapid and functional recovery. Oral and maxillofacial oncological surgery requires specific precision instruments and techniques. The anatomy of the oral cavity is complex and contains important vasculature and innervation. Moreover, access to the oral cavity is limited and the soft tissues there must be handled delicately.

In this sense, piezoelectric bone surgery tools generate a specific cutting frequency for intervening the bone that does not affect soft tissues, allow precise cuts to be made by optimally adapting to difficult locations, do not damage the mucosa, reduce bleeding, and minimize the risk of postoperative swelling.

Malignant neoplasms have a high capacity for bone invasion and can travel to other locations (metastasis).

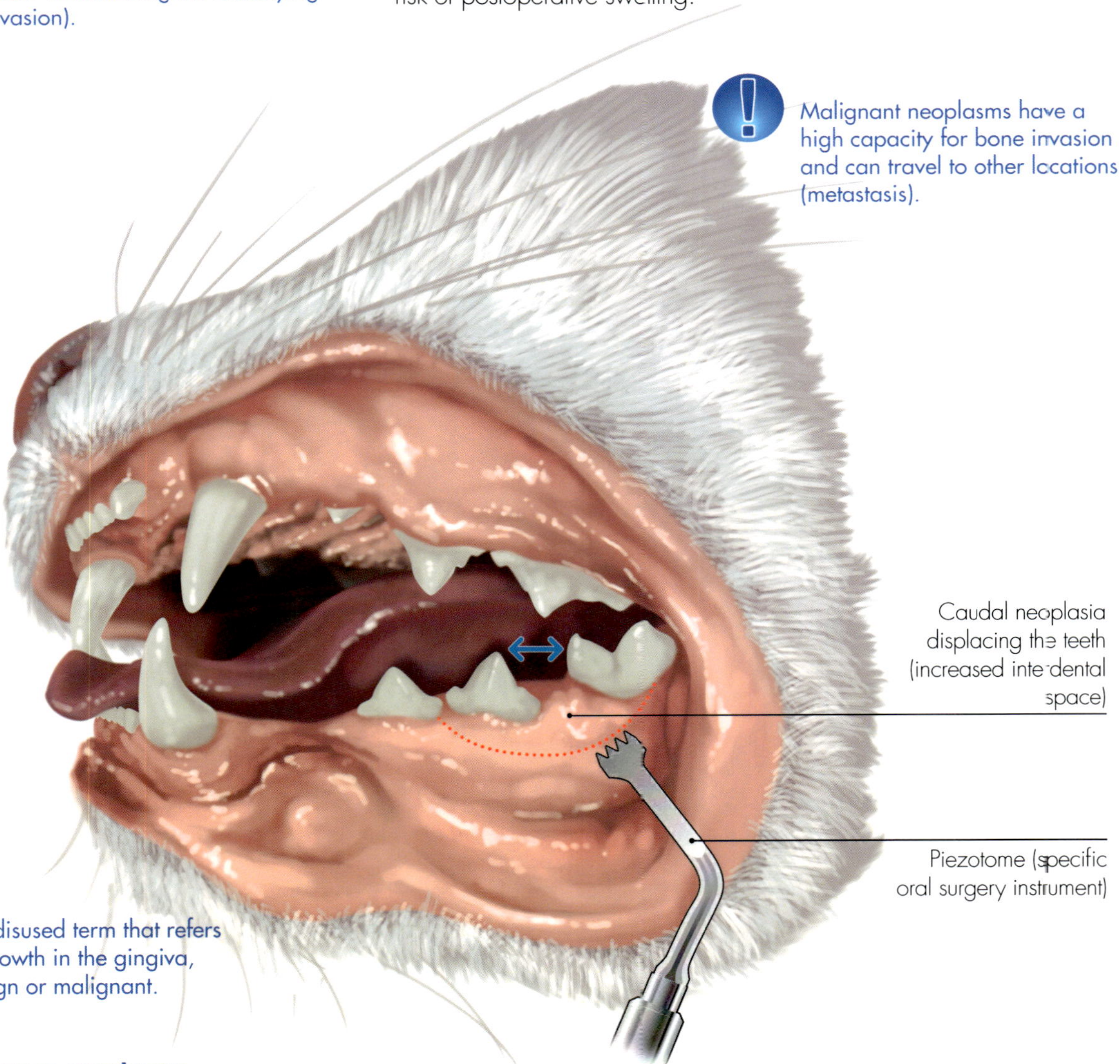

"Epulis" is a disused term that refers to any overgrowth in the gingiva, whether benign or malignant.

Most common neoplasms

Odontogenic	Nonodontogenic
Acanthomatous ameloblastoma	Malignant melanoma
Peripheral odontogenic fibroma	Squamous cell carcinoma
Feline inductive odontogenic tumor	Fibrosarcoma

37 Salivary gland alterations

Salivary glands are responsible for the production of saliva, whose function is to lubricate and protect the oral mucosa. They are classified as major and minor:

- Major: Zygomatic, parotid, mandibular, and sublingual (monostomatic and polystomatic portions).
- Minor: Labial, lingual, and palatine (molar in cats).

Salivary glands in dogs

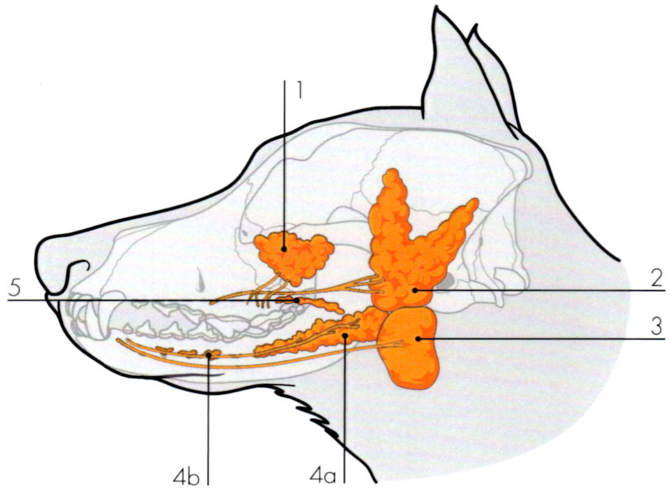

1. Zygomatic gland
2. Parotid gland
3. Mandibular gland

4a. Monostomatic sublingual gland
4b. Polystomatic sublingual gland
5. Palatine gland

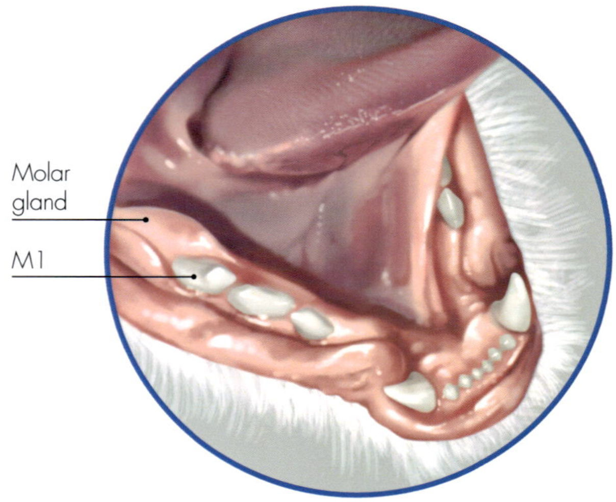

Cats have a molar salivary gland located in the membranous molar pad lingual to the mandibular first molar.

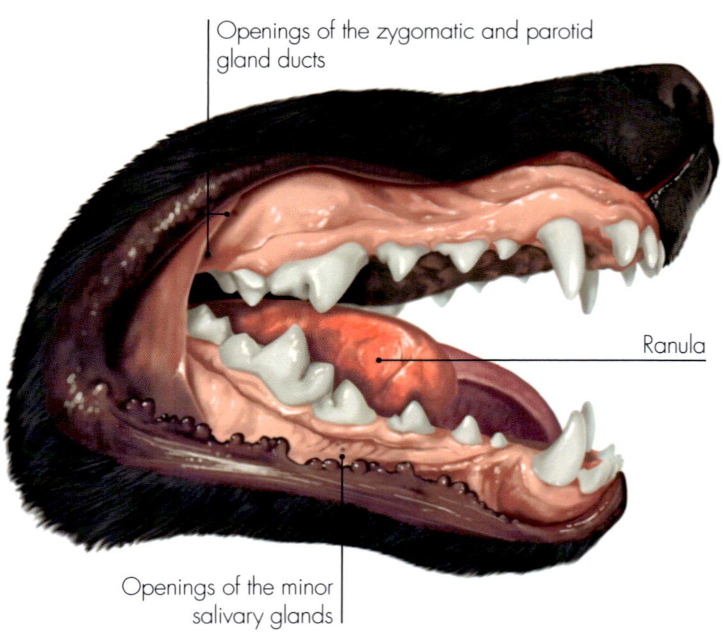

Most common alterations

- **Sialocele:** Accumulation of saliva due to the rupture of a salivary gland or its ducts.
- **Ranula:** Sialocele located under the tongue.
- **Sialolith:** Mineralization (stone) that forms inside a gland or its duct.

Diagnosis of salivary gland pathology

- Contrast radiography: sialography. It is useful when a foreign body or sialolith is suspected.
- Computed tomography (CT) and magnetic resonance imaging (MRI). Current diagnostic methods allow to find the exact location of the problem and help with planning the surgical treatment procedure.

38 Local anesthesia: Blocks

Anesthetic blocks provide better anesthesia and analgesia in painful procedures such as dental extractions or any other oral cavity surgery. They reduce the requirements for inhalation and intravenous anesthetic drugs and contribute to better recovery after surgery by controlling post-operative pain.

1. Inferior alveolar nerve block

Recommended technique for dental extractions.

In the mandibular foramen. An intraoral approach is also possible.

Anesthetized area: Bone, soft tissues, and all the teeth of the mandible.

2. Maxillary nerve block

Recommended technique for dental extractions.

Anesthetized area: Lip and incisors from the anesthetized side rostrally, plus the fourth premolar, molars, and palate.

3. Infraorbital nerve block

In the maxillary foramen.

Anesthetized area: Rostral part of the lip and the incisors, canines, and premolars on the anesthetized side up to the fourth premolar.

4. Middle mental nerve block

In the middle mental foramen.

Anesthetized area: Lip, mucosa, and gingiva.

Negative aspiration should always be performed to avoid accidental intravenous injection.

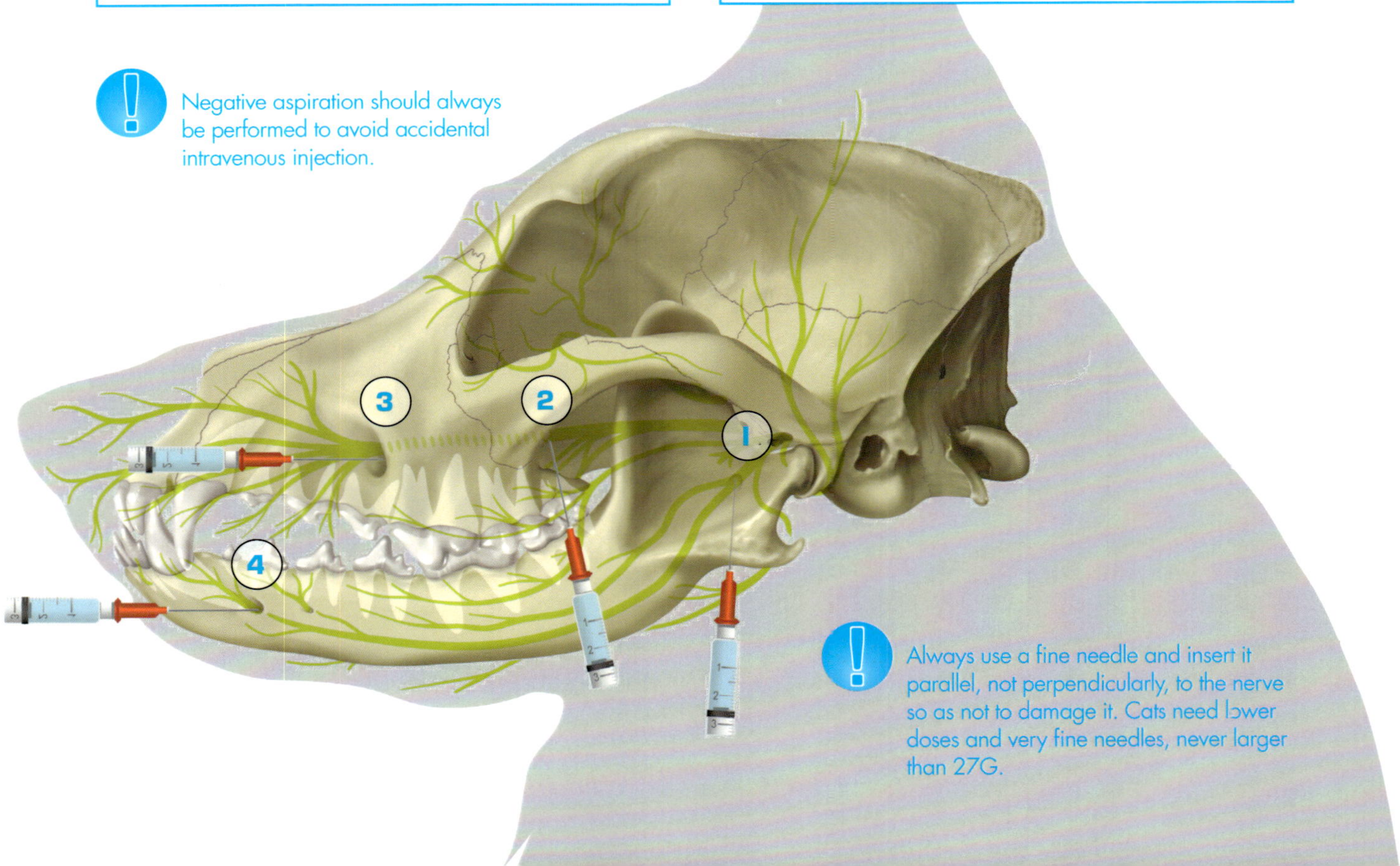

Always use a fine needle and insert it parallel, not perpendicularly, to the nerve so as not to damage it. Cats need lower doses and very fine needles, never larger than 27G.

39 Dental extractions

Tooth extraction (exodontics) is one of the most frequent procedures carried out in small animal practice. Both simple extractions and open flap extractions are surgical techniques that require the use of appropriate instrumentation and proper training.

General considerations

The owner must give consent for dental extractions and the use of both general anesthesia and local anesthetic blocks are required because these surgical procedures are painful.

Recovery is very good if appropriate postoperative analgesia is provided. The dog or cat will be able to eat their usual food even more comfortably than before treatment, because they will feel relief from elimination of the infection and alleviation of pain.

Canines and carnassial teeth

The extraction of large teeth (canines and carnassial teeth) requires the use of appropriate surgical techniques and is often referred to a dental specialist, because specific instruments are needed for odontosection and subsequent extraction of multirooted teeth.

No dental procedures should be performed under sedation (recommendations of the WSAVA, EVDC, and AVDC).

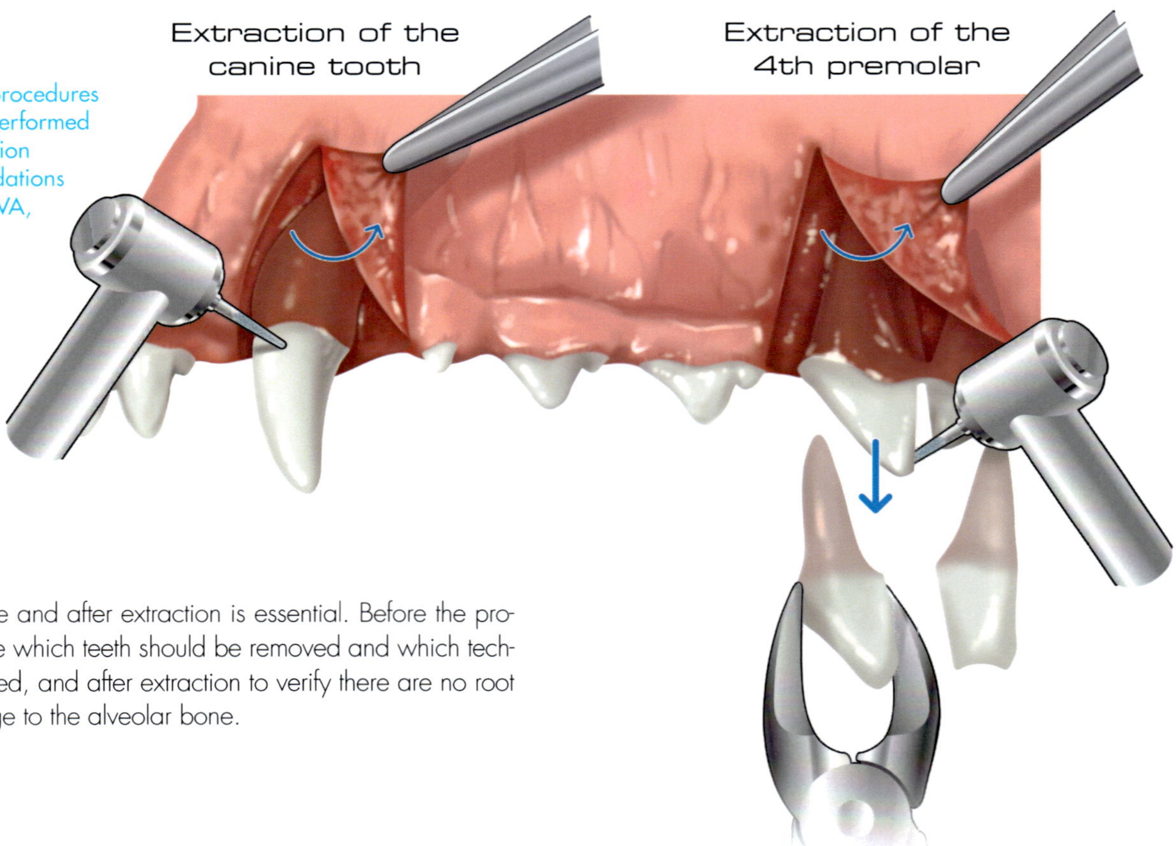

Radiography before and after extraction is essential. Before the procedure to determine which teeth should be removed and which technique should be used, and after extraction to verify there are no root remnants or damage to the alveolar bone.

Indications

- Advanced periodontal disease.
- Moderate periodontal disease in cases where the owner cannot perform maintenance hygiene (daily tooth brushing).
- Tooth resorption.
- Dental fractures (if endodontics cannot be performed).
- Pulp pathologies (if endodontics cannot be performed).
- Feline and canine stomatitis.
- Persistent deciduous teeth.
- Supernumerary teeth that interfere with occlusion or cause crowding.
- Malocclusion that cannot be corrected by orthodontics.

40 Advanced periodontal treatment

Treatment of moderate and severe periodontal disease is performed by applying surgical techniques. When periodontal pockets are deep (more than 4–5 mm, depending on the size of the animal and tooth type), surgical exposure improves access to the roots for root scaling and removal of inflamed and infected tissue, which helps regenerate tooth support.

Open periodontal treatment

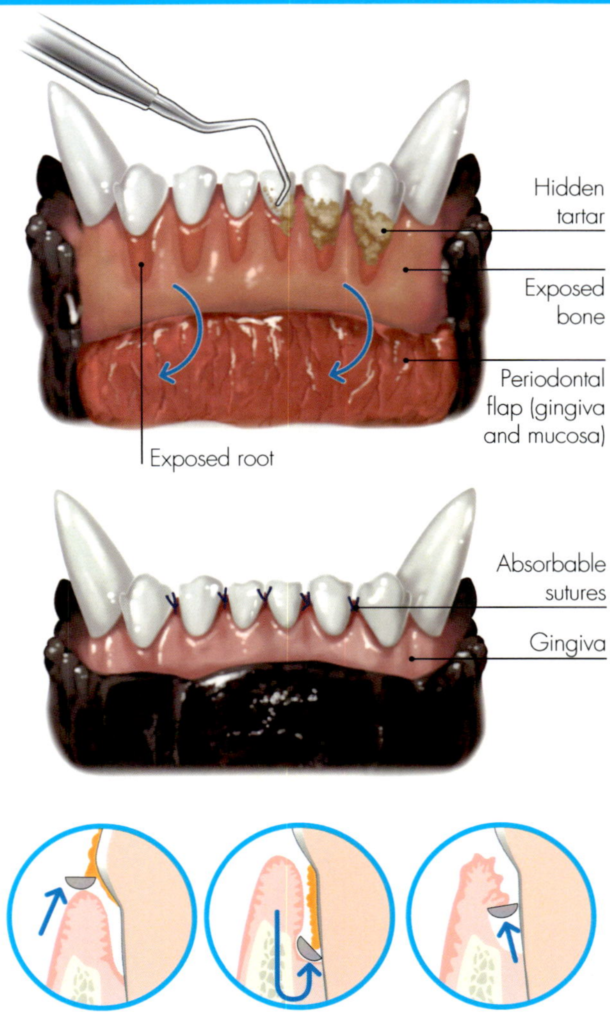

- Surgical exposure of the roots facilitates treatment.
- After root scaling and planing, the gingival contour is restored by suturing the flap.
- These techniques should be performed by a specialist.

Guided tissue regeneration

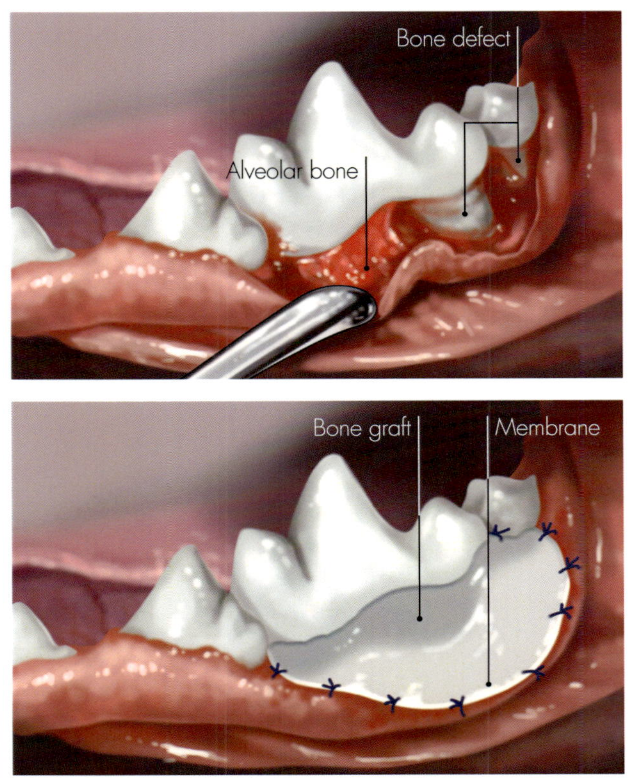

- The defect must be meticulously cleaned prior to the introduction of any material.
- Bone graft or biomaterial and membrane.
- The treatment objective is regeneration of the tissues supporting the tooth by using membranes, to prevent epithelial migration, and bone grafts to fill the defect.

! Proof that the owner has the ability to ensure a good daily tooth brushing routine is required; otherwise, this type of periodontal surgery is contraindicated (see Sheet 19).

41 Gingivectomy

Gingival overgrowth is frequent in some predisposed breeds such as the West Highland White Terrier. It is also associated with medical treatments, hormonal changes, and chronic gingivitis.

Gingival hyperplasia is one of the most common benign causes of gingival enlargement, but any type of overgrowth detected should be biopsied to rule out the presence of other oral neoplasms.

Some young cats suffer from a process of gingival enlargement called juvenile gingivitis.

Gingivectomy is contraindicated when there is less than 2 mm of attached gingiva or when bone loss extends beyond the mucogingival junction.

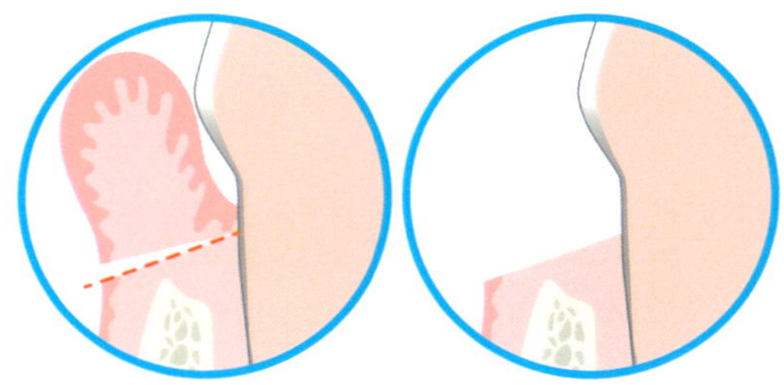

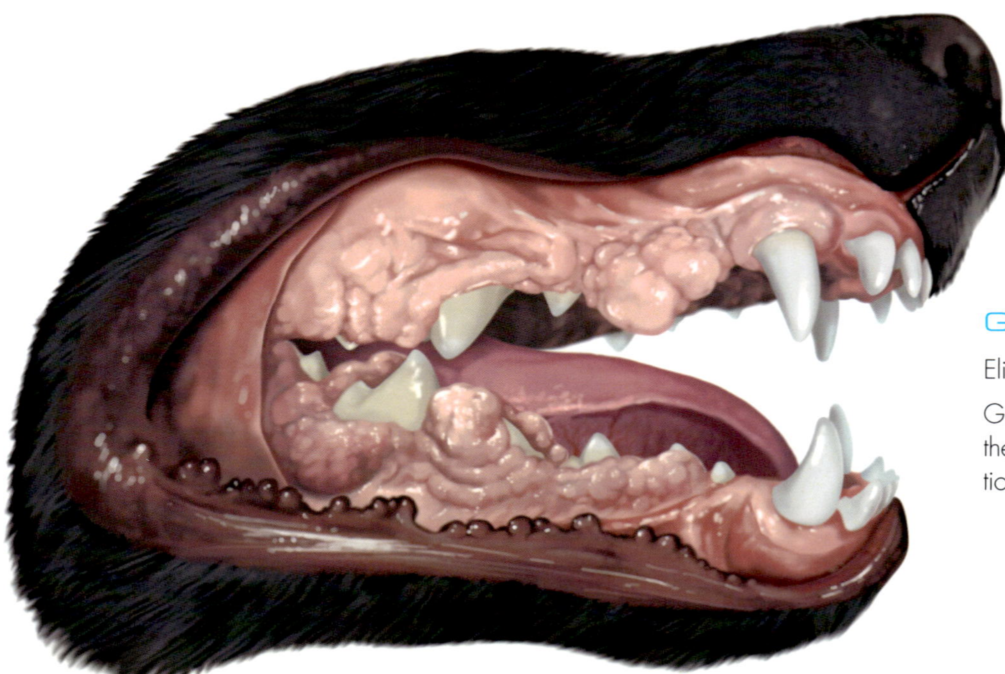

Gingivectomy

Elimination of excess gingiva.

Gingival overgrowth covering part of the tooth crown favors the accumulation of plaque and food debris.

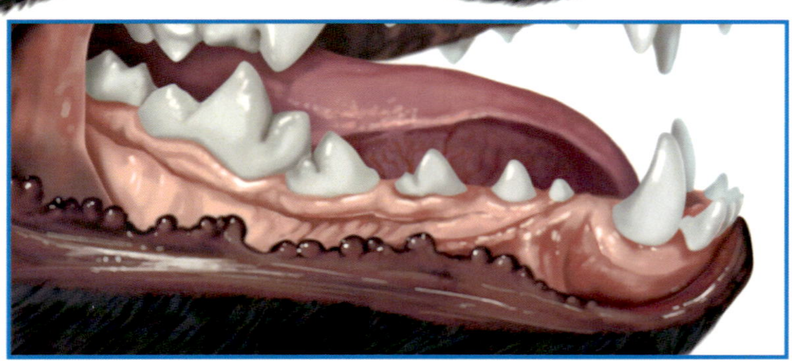

Gingivoplasty

Final treatment to restore a normal gingival contour.

Intraoral radiography is essential to determine the extent of bone loss.

42 Alternatives to extraction: Endodontics

The pulp cavity houses the pulp tissue that nourishes and innervates the tooth. Dental vitality can be compromised because of trauma or fractures exposing the pulp and leading to infection.

Endodontics is a good alternative to extraction because it preserves the tooth and, therefore, its function, even if it has lost vitality.

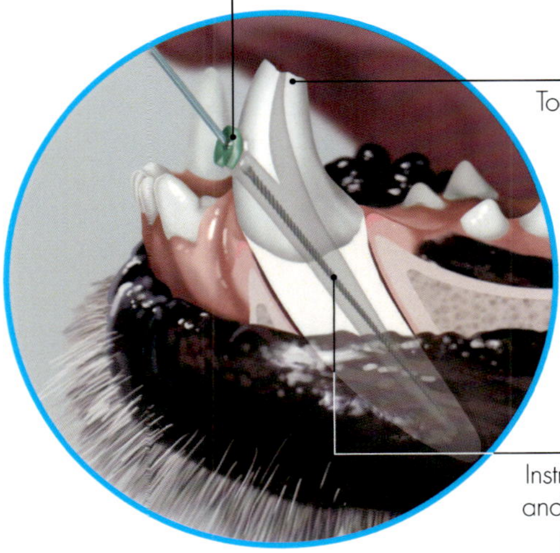

Features

Endodontics involves cleaning and disinfecting the root canal, obturating the canal with biocompatible materials, and restoring the access points.

This treatment requires radiographic follow-up at 6 months and annual revision.

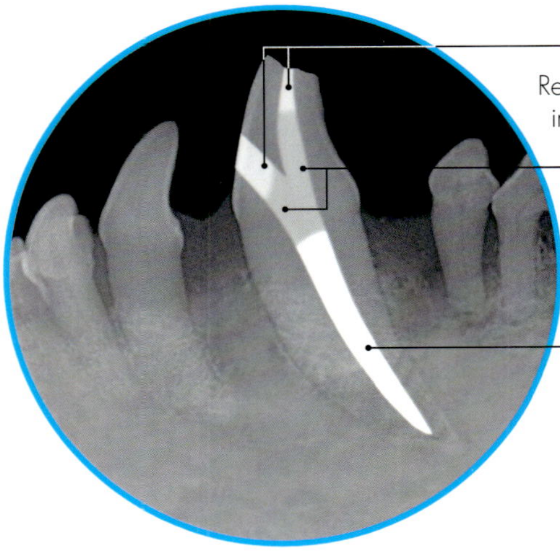

Advantages over extraction

- It avoids dental extraction and its associated complications such as the risk of mandibular fracture (see Sheet 39).
- The facial structure and tooth function are maintained.
- It prevents the lip entrapment that occurs in some cases after extraction of the maxillary canine (see Sheet 39), as well as tongue drooping and excessive drooling.

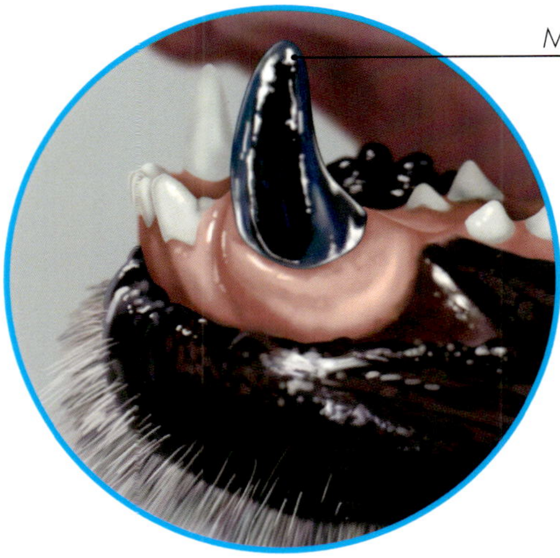

Some cases also benefit from the placement of a metal cap or crown to protect the restoration and prevent the tooth from fracturing again.

43 Vital pulp therapy

Vital pulp therapy consists of removing only a portion of the pulp tissue and then applying a treatment that stimulates healing and repair by creating dentinal bridges. This allows the tooth to stay vital and continue to mature. Young animals with immature teeth generally have a better prognosis with this type of treatment.

Indications

Recent (less than 48 hours) dental fractures, and crown reduction in cases of malocclusion that causes tissue damage and cannot be corrected by orthodontics.

Radiological monitoring is essential to assess tooth maturation.

Traumatic fracture

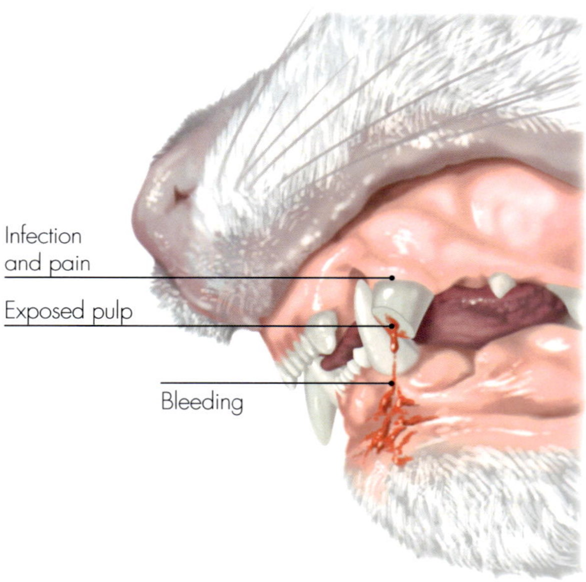

A dental fracture with pulp exposure is very painful. At first there is bleeding and the pulp is reddened, but then the bleeding disappears and may go unnoticed by the owner. The animal may show no clinical signs and in fact, if the owner was not present when the trauma occurred, it usually goes unnoticed.

Crown reduction in malocclusion cases

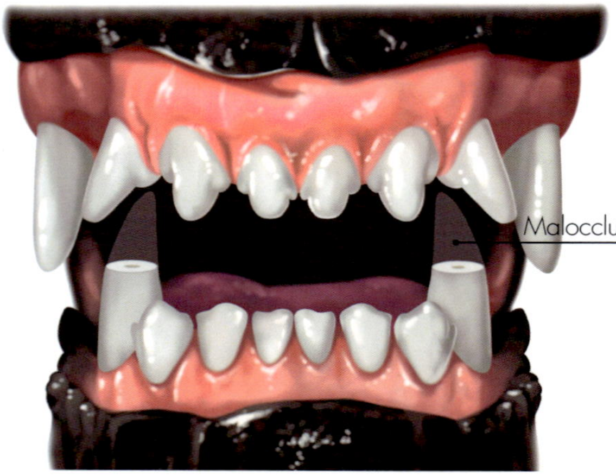

This technique is performed under sterile conditions (as opposed to cases with fractures), and so the success rate is higher.

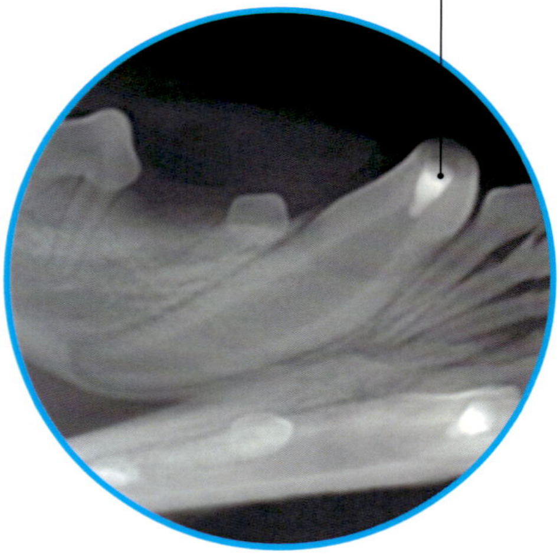

Dental fractures are painful and should be referred to a specialist as soon as possible. To maintain tooth vitality, treatment should be started within 48 hours of trauma.

44 Orthodontic solutions

Orthodontics is the branch of dentistry that deals with correcting the position of the teeth by using various devices and mechanisms. The objective of these interventions is to give the animal a comfortable and functional bite. For ethical reasons, purely aesthetic alterations do not require treatment. In addition, animals with malocclusion of genetic origin should not be bred.

Orthodontic solutions are less invasive than tooth extractions and avoid the complications associated with extractions of large teeth such as canines and carnassial teeth (see Sheet 39).

Disadvantages

- This technique requires several anesthetic procedures.
- Orthodontic treatments should be performed by a specialist.
- The owner's collaboration regarding daily oral hygiene and periodic checkups is required.

Correction with an acrylic inclined plane

An example of fixed passive orthodontics commonly used to correct mandibular canine linguoversion (see Sheet 9). The canines slowly move back to their normal position when the dog's mouth is closed. Treatments usually only last for a short period (6–8 weeks).

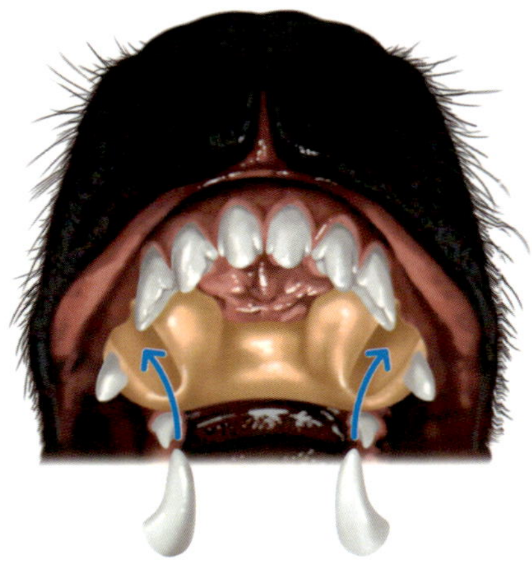

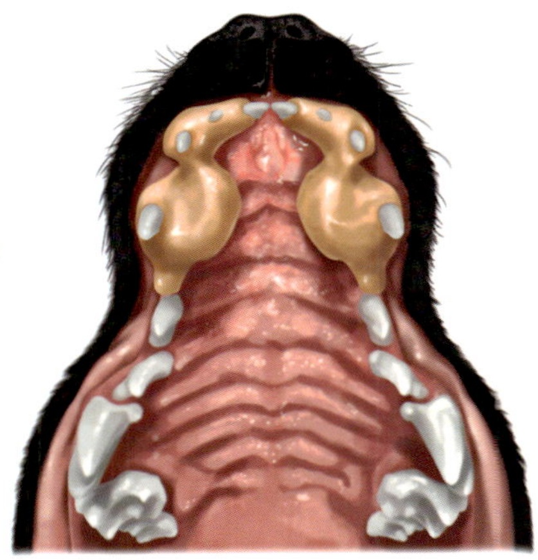

Correction with braces and an elastic chain

An example of active orthodontics indicated for the correction of a mesially displaced maxillary canine. The elastic chain is changed periodically to achieve tooth movement.

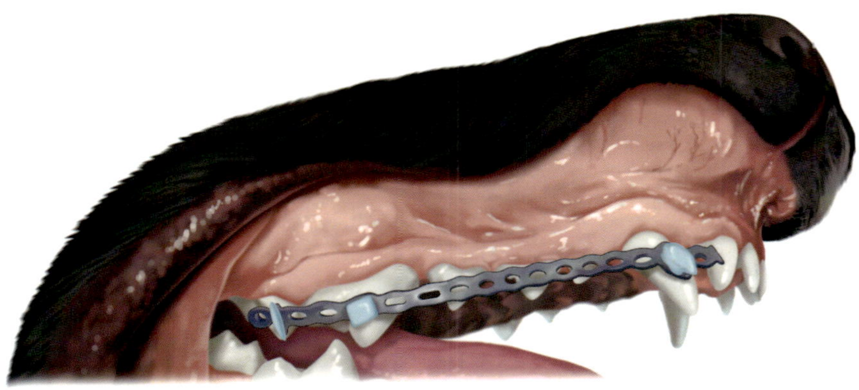

45 Maxillofacial trauma

Maxillofacial trauma is very common in small animals as the result of road traffic accidents, falls from a height, and fights with other animals. In addition, small-sized breed dogs with advanced periodontitis are prone to pathological fractures secondary to bone loss (see Sheet 17).

The complications associated with repair of these fractures by using conventional screws and osteosynthesis plates are the result of the specific characteristics of the bones of the face: the teeth occupy most of the jawbone, and the mandibular canal houses vessels and nerves that must not be damaged.

Diagnosis

- Combination of intraoral radiography and computed tomography (CT).
- Conventional skull radiographs are of little use because of the presence of overlapping structures.
- The most appropriate diagnostic method is CT, as it is the easiest way to detect the multiple fractures that usually occur in maxillofacial trauma and are often not evident upon examination.

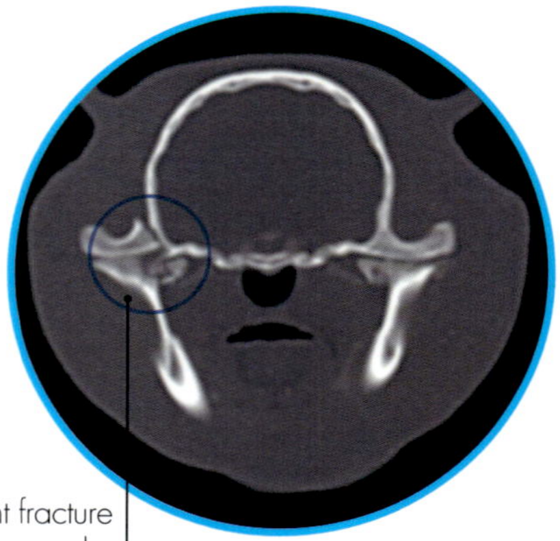

Temporomandibular joint fracture seen by computed tomography

Intraoral fixation with an acrylic splint reinforced with cerclage wire

Intraoral fixation methods are minimally invasive and promote rapid patient recovery. In addition, they avoid damaging the vasculature and innervation of the face and facilitate the maintenance of normal occlusion.

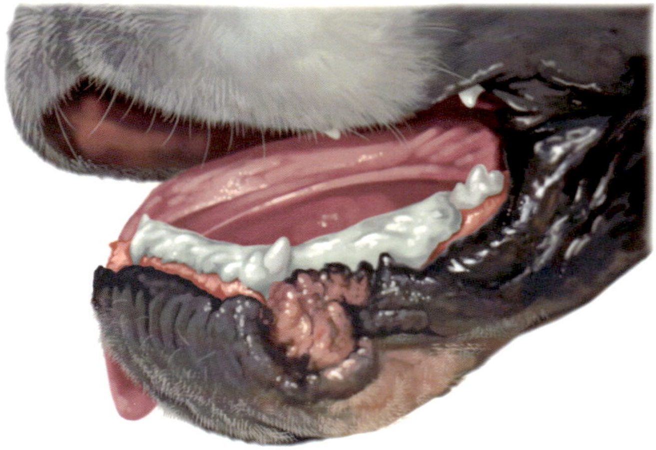

Maxillomandibular fixation

It maintains normal occlusion with the mouth half open so that the animal can eat a liquid diet.

Esophagostomy tube placement is recommended to administer medication and ensure adequate food intake.

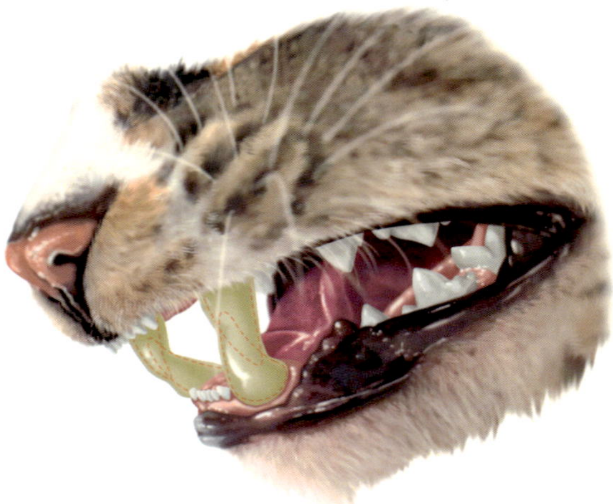

46 Custom-made adhesive tape muzzles

This is an economical and effective method to stabilize the mouth of patients with maxillofacial trauma, especially as an initial means of stabilization until surgery or referral to a specialist is possible.

Nylon muzzles commercially available in different sizes can also be used.

These muzzles are used to stabilize the fracture and keep the mouth closed in order to preserve interdigitation of the teeth. Some slack must be allowed for the animal to reach its tongue out to drink water or eat a liquid diet.

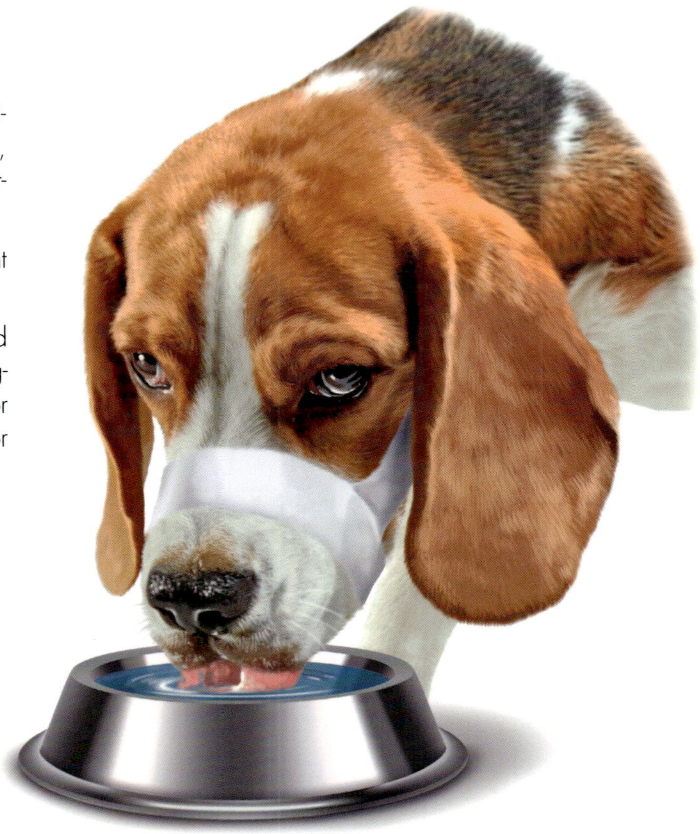

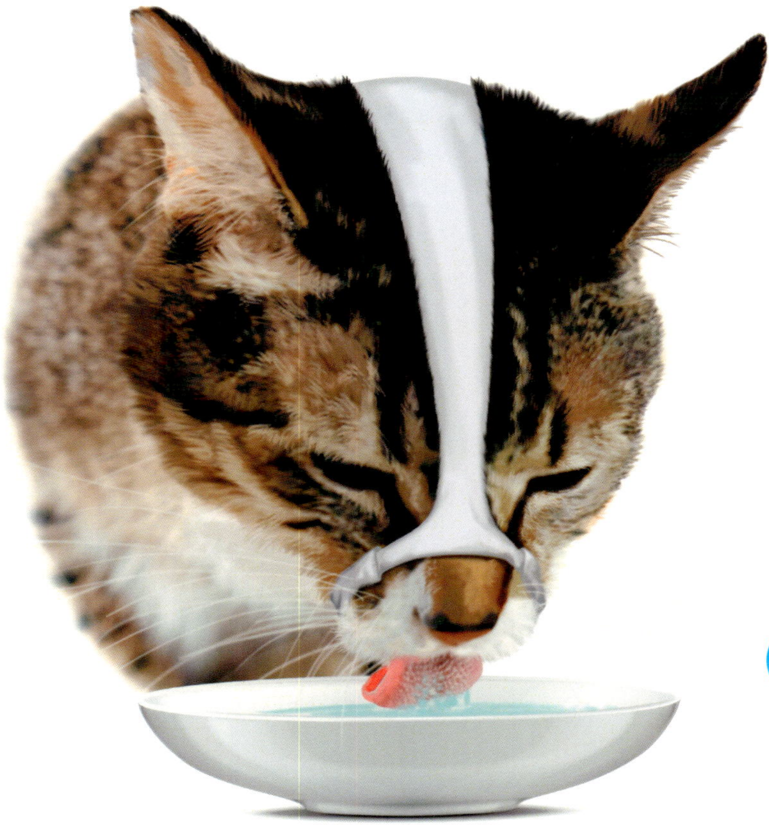

Key points

- In-house custom fabrication allows for adjustment to differences in the size of each patient's skull.
- Several equal units should be created so the owner can replace the muzzle when it is wet or dirty, thereby avoiding the appearance of dermatitis.

These muzzles can serve as the sole treatment in puppies and young adults with nondisplaced mandibular fractures.